Caring for the Displaced and Uninsured

Caring for the Displaced and Uninsured

Clinical Case Studies in Nursing & Healthcare

Leslie Neal-Boylan
Mansfield Kaseman Health Clinic
Rockville, MD
USA

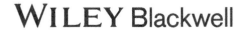

Registered Offices
John Wiley & Sons, Inc., 111 River Street, Hoboken, NJ 07030, USA
John Wiley & Sons Ltd, The Atrium, Southern Gate, Chichester, West Sussex, PO19 8SQ, UK

Editorial Office
9600 Garsington Road, Oxford, OX4 2DQ, UK

For details of our global editorial offices, customer services, and more information about Wiley products, visit us at www.wiley.com.

Wiley also publishes its books in a variety of electronic formats and by print-on-demand. Some content that appears in standard print versions of this book may not be available in other formats.

Library of Congress Cataloging-in-Publication Data Applied for
Paperback: 9781119866039

Cover Design: Wiley
Cover Image: © Creative-Touch/Getty Images

Set in 9.5/12.5pt STIXTwoText by Straive, Pondicherry, India
SKY10036236_092922

Contents

Acknowledgments

This book is dedicated to the wonderful patients from all over the world who've challenged my mind and enriched my soul. They've taught me the petty trials of life are nothing when one is struggling for basic survival. They've helped me understand of how little importance are so many things with which privileged Americans concern themselves. We take for granted food, clothing, shelter, employment, healthcare, safety, and companionship, although most of the rest of the world goes without at least one of these things every day. These patients are incredibly resilient; many describe themselves as happy despite their struggles. Those who are unhappy are legitimately so based on the profound difficulties they've endured. Together, we face their health care challenges. We also laugh and cry and share. I'm so grateful to be a small part of their lives.

This book is also dedicated to the incredible volunteers without whom I could not do my work. The volunteer healthcare providers, students, retirees, and others who just want to help are amazing people who give their time and talents (and sometimes their treasure) to help us and our patients.

Preface

This book emerged from my clinical practice as the only full-time healthcare provider in a small clinic for uninsured, mostly immigrant patients. I had worked in community clinics before as well as in private practice, student health, and urgent care. Despite many years of experience as a nurse and a nurse practitioner, I was unprepared for the beyond-clinical aspects of this type of practice.

The case studies within this book focus on the issues faced primarily by patients who are uninsured, self-pay, or are visiting from their home countries. The latter may be insured in their home countries but are not insured in the United States. Patients who have Medicaid or Medicare are also included because they have access to different, not always better, resources than those who are uninsured. Self-pay patients are typically those who make too much money to be eligible for resources available to the uninsured but either do not make enough money to purchase insurance or prefer not to do so.

Each clinic of this type is different depending on their structure and financial support. However, working with the uninsured, particularly immigrants, to provide them timely and high-quality healthcare with minimal resources is consistent across the board.

This book is not intended to be paternalistic or dictate how providers should approach people from other countries, ethnicities, races, or cultures. Rather, the goal is to share strategies that have proved useful and have assisted both patients and providers to have a comfortable, high-quality primary care clinic experience. The names of the home countries from which these patients came to the United States are not provided, partly to protect patient anonymity and partly to preclude the temptation to group all people from one place as looking, acting, or responding in the same way. Patients, regardless of from where they originate or where they live, remain individuals and should always be treated as such without preconceived assumptions. However, it is helpful for the clinician to think in broader terms when treating immigrant and/or uninsured patients beyond how we are taught to approach patients who have been raised in the United States.

I hope this book emphasizes the ongoing disparities in healthcare access for uninsured, especially immigrant, patients and the urgent need to offer high-quality, equitable, affordable care to everyone. This book offers tips for providers to provide quality healthcare within the parameters that currently exist.

While the cases are clinical and take place in a primary care setting, the focus is less on the clinical diagnosis and treatment than on how diagnosis and treatment are achieved for patients with little to no financial resources. Federally Qualified Health Centers (FQHCs) tend to have more resources for patients than do smaller clinics that depend on state or local funding and grants. The patients in these cases are from the latter.

Clinicians working in these clinics are at the heart of patient care. The patients we serve frequently arrive in the United States without previous medical care or with minimal previous healthcare. If they received healthcare, it may be primitive compared to the cutting-edge medical care in the United States. Many patients have never had dental care or vision screening. Both are sources of potential impairments and pain.

The clinic is a lifeline and a conduit to healthcare and resources that may help patients with food, housing, and bill paying. Advocacy is the priority because many of these patients would not otherwise have healthcare unless they went to urgent care clinics or the emergency department for which they would have to pay, even with payment plans, much more than they pay at these clinics.

Deference and respect are important attributes for the clinician working in any health care setting; however, many of these patients have already experienced significant hardship, discrimination, and sometimes torture in their own countries, while traveling to the United States, or once here. Not only can the clinician in this setting set the tone by representing Americans in a good light but they engender patient trust by treating them deferentially and respectfully.

Visits in these clinics require more time than in private clinics. Not only do new patients or patients returning after several years require extensive histories and physical exams because they may not have had any medical care for a long time, if at all, but also because they may have multiple comorbidities, some of which can be very serious.

Patients may return to the clinic only when they are worried or have a new problem because they cannot afford the visit or the time away from work. Many patients work in hourly wage jobs and may lose their jobs if they take time off. Their work is often very physically demanding, such as house cleaning, child care, housekeeping, restaurant kitchen work, landscaping, or various types of construction work. They often present with musculoskeletal complaints or specific concerns arising from their work. Many work in multiple jobs in addition to caring for their children and/or other family members or friends. It is important that the clinician be generous with notes for work that allow a couple of days off to rest or days off from heavy lifting or other physical work. Sometimes, rest is all the patient needs to feel better.

Some patients live in shelters or basements or with their employers. They may be exploited by landlords or employers and are largely unaware of "how things are done" in the United States, expecting to have to bribe officials or wait in long lines for food.

This is healthcare at its most basic and its most complicated. It is basic because sometimes all that is needed is rest and a mild analgesic. It is complicated when the patient needs much more, but rest and an analgesic are all they can access. The clinician is constantly challenged to get patients what they need regardless of the barriers. This requires the clinician to be creative and to develop strong relationships with outside providers and volunteer specialists. "Curbside consultations" are frequently necessary to treat patients who cannot get to or afford specialty care.

Patients may not know the names of their conditions or the medicines they have been given, if they received any in the past. In addition, they may receive medicines from a neighborhood Latin store or from friends or have them sent from their home countries with or without a prescription. The ingredients of the medicine may be unclear or untested. Patients may maintain a televisit relationship with a provider in their home country. Many use herbs, cupping, or other alternative treatments. Patients rarely bring documentation from health visits in their home country or with televisit providers. It is frequently necessary to "start from scratch."

Patients may take their medicines sporadically to save money and frequently think they are done with their medicines when the prescription ends. They do not always know they need to return to the clinic periodically to be rechecked and receive refills. They may not be aware the prescription allows for a refill or how to obtain the refill. If they are aware but don't have the money to pay for the refill, they may wait so long to refill the medication that the prescription has expired. Some patients share their medications with friends or family members who cannot get to the clinic.

Many clinics provide free medications based on evidence showing the patient meets a certain federal poverty level. Medicare, Medicaid, and self-pay patients are not typically eligible for these free medications. Some clinics may be able to afford to give patients some free or low-cost immunizations, but frequently patients must get vaccinations at local pharmacies. Vaccinations can be unaffordable without insurance. Patients may not get blood work or other tests due to financial concerns and may be reluctant to or unaware they can ask for an installment plan.

Volunteers are integral to the clinic. The clinic budget is typically too low to hire as many staff as needed to comfortably run the clinic. Volunteer healthcare providers are especially important because their presence in person or in a televisit increases patient access to specialty care, such as endocrinology, pulmonology, and gastroenterology. Volunteers who help at reception and the front desk can relieve paid staff from answering phones and data entry. Some translators are people who volunteer their time or are premedical or nursing students who want experience in a community clinic.

Translators are necessary in these clinics; in person is preferred. The rapport developed between translator and patient is important to the patient–provider relationship. Patients may tell translators details they do not tell the provider, feeling a greater degree of comfort with someone who speaks their own language. If possible, it is ideal for the provider to speak the patient's language or at least make an effort to do so. However, patients come from all over the world to these clinics. Phone interpreter access can be sporadic and is not as effective as in-person translation. Translators are frequently volunteers without experience in professional translation. Training is necessary because visits can go off course if the translator translates more than the provider has said. Translators may say words differently despite speaking the same language. They should always use the formal version of language rather than the informal version and should refrain from asking questions the provider had not asked. There is a fine line between having a rapport with the patient and becoming too informal. Patients have different levels of education. It is important that translators know they may have to simplify their translation for certain patients. Some translators will feel compelled to give medical advice, especially if they have worked in healthcare or are medical or nursing students. It is necessary for them to separate their role as translator from their role as healthcare provider.

In addition to the deference and respect mentioned above, awareness of what people from other cultures might find offensive is an important attribute of the clinician. Patients from other cultures may be very religious and might be offended if asked if they use birth control, if they have sexual intercourse with someone of their same gender, or if they have ever had a sexually transmitted infection. Naturally, the clinician must obtain a thorough history, and these questions are important. However, sensitivity is especially important because the patient may never have been asked these questions before. Save the questions for a later visit, if possible, once there is a bond of trust with the clinician.

Many of the issues discussed in these cases appear in multiple cases; however, for the sake of organization, the cases have been divided into categories. The "resolutions" of each case are entitled "dilemmas and decisions" rather than "resolutions" because the clinical aspects of the cases are not necessarily resolved in each instance. The "pearl" at the end of each case is an attempt to offer tips and strategies to consider if working with patients with similar backgrounds and/or presentations.

The best way to use the book is to read the case presentation, respond to the critical thinking questions, and then review the "dilemmas and decisions" section for that case. Keep in mind the focus of the book is on caring for these populations in an environment of limited resources. Much more could be done for each patient if the person had the financial ability to pursue other options.

Part I

Cases

1

Family Issues

Evangeline

HPI: Evangeline is a 64-year-old female new patient diagnosed with DM and HTN who has not taken her medications for six months. She works as a housekeeper for three young children. She has five grown children who live in the Philippines. She is trying to earn enough money to go back there. Evangeline is a widow. She says she feels generally well other than intermittent dizziness. Her last medical visit was one year ago in the Middle East.

Medications:

Not taking metformin HCL 500 mg 1 tablet with a meal daily.

Medical/Surgical History:

Diabetes mellitus.
Hypertension.
Stroke, unknown type or date. Evangeline denies residual effects.

FMH:

Family history unknown.
Oldest daughter has DMT2.

Caring for the Displaced and Uninsured: Clinical Case Studies in Nursing & Healthcare, First Edition. Leslie Neal-Boylan.
© 2023 John Wiley & Sons Ltd. Published 2023 by John Wiley & Sons Ltd.

SH:

Denies use of tobacco or recreational drugs. Drinks one 12-oz beer/month. Living with employer. Widowed.

OB/GYN History:

Five pregnancies, five NSVD.
Not currently sexually active.
Postmenopausal.
Pap smear: never.
Mammogram: never.

Allergies: NKDA.

ROS:

HEENT: denies headaches, problems with vision. Has full dentures.
Cardiovascular/respiratory: denies chest pain or palpitations. Admits to dizziness and fluid accumulation in the legs. Denies hemoptysis, pain with inspiration, shortness of breath at rest or with exertion.
GI/GU: denies abdominal pain. Denies blood in stool or urine. Denies change in bladder or bowel habits.
Women only: denies breast lump, breast pain, discharge from the breast, vaginal bleeding.
Musculoskeletal: reports occasional left hip and LB pain.
Skin: denies itching, rash, skin lesion(s).
Neurologic: denies tingling/numbness, tremors.
Psychiatric: denies anxiety, depressed mood. Admits to stressors; she drinks water and rests and feeling of stress resolves.

Vitals Signs:

Ht 61 in, Wt 117 lbs, BP 190/96 mmHg, HR 72/min, RR 18/min, Temp 98.4 F, glucose 210.

General Examination:

GENERAL APPEARANCE: alert, well hydrated, in no distress.
EYES: pupils equal, round, reactive to light and accommodation, extraocular movement intact.
EARS: tympanic membrane intact, clear.
ORAL: mucosa moist, full dentures.

NECK/THYROID: no jugular venous distention, no thyroid nodules, no thyromegaly, thyroid nontender.

SKIN: warm and dry.

HEART: S1, S2 normal, regular rate and rhythm, no murmurs, rubs, gallops, no clicks.

LUNGS: clear to auscultation bilaterally.

ABDOMEN: bowel sounds present, soft, nontender, nondistended, no hepatosplenomegaly, no guarding or rigidity.

BACK: normal exam of spine, spine nontender to palpation, full range of motion.

MUSCULOSKELETAL: cervical spine normal, full range of motion, full range of motion of the hip, lumbosacral spine normal, no swelling or deformity.

EXTREMITIES: full range of motion, good capillary refill in nail beds, no clubbing, cyanosis, or edema.

PERIPHERAL PULSES: 2+ dorsalis pedis, 2+ posterior tibial, 2+ radial.

NEUROLOGIC: nonfocal, alert and oriented, cerebellar function normal, cognitive exam grossly normal, cooperative with exam, deep tendon reflexes 2+ symmetrical, motor strength normal upper and lower extremities, neck supple, no rigidity, no tremor.

PSYCHIATRIC: alert, oriented, cognitive function intact, cooperative with exam, good eye contact, judgment and insight good, speech clear, thought content without suicidal ideation, delusions.

FOOT EXAM: sensory testing performed: sensations diminished. Sensory and motor testing performed: strength normal, pedal pulses are 2+. Visual inspection: normal.

Critical Thinking:

1) What are the major concerns in this case?
2) What is your plan for Evangeline?
3) What teaching is appropriate at this time?

Florence

HPI: Florence, a 45-year-old female, reports pain in the third digit of her right hand shooting up toward her right shoulder × one week. She denies hearing any clicking but does feel a locking sensation when she tries to flex the finger. She is unable to fully flex the digit and has pain during flexion and extension. She denies trauma, heavy lifting, wound or insect/human bite, numbness, tingling, fever, or chills. Florence also reports pain in her right elbow, numbness/tingling in BL wrists/hands, mid LBP, and BL hip pain × 1 month. She works cleaning houses. She denies heavy lifting. She sleeps with her right arm extended on a pillow. She denies trauma.

Medications:

Atorvastatin calcium 20 mg tablet, 1 tablet once a day.
Medical/Surgical History:
Hyperlipidemia.

FMH:

Parents, siblings, and children are alive and well.

SH:

Denies use of tobacco, alcohol, or recreational drugs. Married, works full time cleaning houses.

Vital Signs:

Ht 61.5 in, Wt 154 lbs, BP 110/68 mmHg, HR 72/min, RR 16/min, Temp 96.8 F.

General Examination:

GENERAL APPEARANCE: Florence appears very sad. On questioning, she responds that her father died in her home country 12 days ago. She had not seen him in 14 years. She says she has some family here and she goes to church for consolation. Alert and oriented ×3, well developed, well nourished.
EYES: pupils equal, round, reactive to light and accommodation, extraocular movement intact.
SKIN: warm and dry, no erythema, cyanosis, pallor, mottling, ecchymosis or streaking of skin of hands.
HEART: S1, S2 normal, regular rate and rhythm, no murmurs, rubs, gallops, no clicks.
LUNGS: clear to auscultation bilaterally.

MUSCULOSKELETAL: Pt is unable to fully flex third digit right hand. She can extend her finger but with moderate pain. The third digit is significantly swollen. Pt has + right MCP squeeze. She has decreased strength in her right hand 3/5. No pain on ROM of right wrist. No pain in elbow or shoulder but she does have TTP on her right forearm. UEs DTRs are +1. Negative Phalen's test and negative Tinel's test BL. FROM of trunk, hips, knees without pain, no swelling or deformity.
PERIPHERAL PULSES: 2+ radial, 2+ ulnar.
NEUROLOGIC: nonfocal, alert and oriented.

Critical Thinking:

1) What are the major concerns in this case?
2) What is your plan for Florence?
3) What is appropriate teaching at this time?

Gloria

HPI: Gloria, a 26-year-old African female, presents to the clinic for constipation. She reports she has not had a bowel movement in three days. Her last bowel movement was hard and consisted of small "balls." She denies bleeding. Gloria drinks two glasses of water daily. She describes a diet of mostly plantains, rice, and fufu (fermented casava). She rarely eats vegetables or rice. Gloria reports her mother died yesterday in Africa. She was very close to her mother and had not seen her in many years.

Medications:

None.

Medical/Surgical History:

None.

FMH:

Mother had diabetes mellitus; died yesterday age 58 of the COVID-19 virus. Mother lived in Gloria's home country. Father died at age 35 of unknown causes. No siblings. Gloria has three children who are alive and well. Husband is alive and well.

SH:

Married, lives with husband, children, and three nieces and nephews. Lives in a small apartment; unemployed. Denies use of tobacco, alcohol, recreational drugs.

Vital Signs:

Ht 56 in, Wt 175 lbs, BP 100/70 mmHg, HR 72 /min, RR 14 /min, Temp 97.7 F.

General Examination:

GENERAL APPEARANCE: alert and oriented ×3, crying.
EYES: pupils equal, round, reactive to light and accommodation.
SKIN: warm and dry.
HEART: S1, S2 normal, regular rate and rhythm, no murmurs, rubs, gallops, no clicks.
LUNGS: clear to auscultation bilaterally.
ABDOMEN: BS normoactive, soft, NT, no HSM, no guarding.
EXTREMITIES: good capillary refill in nail beds, no clubbing, cyanosis, or edema.
PERIPHERAL PULSES: 2+ dorsalis pedis, 2+ posterior tibial, 2+ radial.
NEUROLOGIC: nonfocal, alert and oriented, cognitive exam grossly normal, cooperative with exam, no rigidity, no tremor.
PSYCH: alert, oriented, cognitive function intact, cooperative with exam, good eye contact, speech clear, thought content without suicidal ideation, delusions.

Critical Thinking:

1) What are the major concerns in this case?
2) What is your plan for Gloria?
3) What teaching is appropriate at this time?

2

Medication Issues

Ali

HPI: Ali, a 67-year-old female, presents as a new patient from India. Two weeks ago, she went to the hospital for chest pain. She was diagnosed with syncope. A baby aspirin daily was added to the medication regimen. Her son accompanies her and says that in her home country she was told she had "a pancreas that was drained of water." The son says the diabetes began shortly after the diagnosis. The patient's son asks if something can be done with the pancreas to reverse diabetes. Ali was placed on atorvastatin in the hospital but stopped taking it. She denies signs or symptoms of hypoglycemia. She denies pain, fever, or chills. She refuses a Pap test or mammogram. She does not have a glucometer.

Medications:

Humulin N 100 unit/ml suspension as directed, subcutaneous 40 units in a.m., 26 units in p.m.
Humulin R 100 unit/ml solution as directed, injection 14 units in a.m., 14 units in p.m.
Alendronate sodium 70 mg tablet, 1 tablet orally once a week.
Atorvastatin 40 mg tablets, 40 mg orally once a day.
Vitamin D3 daily.

Caring for the Displaced and Uninsured: Clinical Case Studies in Nursing & Healthcare,
First Edition. Leslie Neal-Boylan.
© 2023 John Wiley & Sons Ltd. Published 2023 by John Wiley & Sons Ltd.

Medical/Surgical History:

Diabetes mellitus type 2.
Osteoporosis.
Hyperlipidemia.
Syncope.

FMH:

Both parents deceased from unknown causes. Siblings and children are
alive and well.

SH:

Denies use of tobacco, alcohol, or recreational drugs. Divorced, lives
with adult son, unemployed.

OB/GYN History:

Seven pregnancies; seven NSVD.
Last Pap smear: 10 years ago, negative.
Last mammogram: 10 years ago, negative.
Menopause: began at age 48.

ROS:

HEENT: denies headaches, problems with vision.
Cardiovascular/respiratory: denies chest pain, syncope, dizziness, fluid
accumulation in the legs, palpitations, pain with inspiration, short-
ness of breath at rest or with exertion.
GI/GU: denies abdominal pain, blood in stool or urine, change in bowel
habits, constipation, difficulty urinating.
Musculoskeletal: denies joint stiffness, painful joints.
Skin: denies dry skin, changing moles, rash.
Neurologic: denies tingling/numbness.
Psychiatric: denies anxiety, depressed mood.

Vital Signs:

Ht 61 in, Wt 138 lbs, BP 168/88, HR 60/min, RR 16/min, Temp 97.2 F.

General Examination:

GENERAL APPEARANCE: alert, well hydrated, in no distress, does not usually make eye contact, defers to daughter.

EYES: pupils equal, round, reactive to light and accommodation, extraocular movement intact.

SKIN: warm and dry.

HEART: S1, S2 normal, regular rate and rhythm, no murmurs, rubs, gallops, no clicks.

LUNGS: clear to auscultation bilaterally.

EXTREMITIES: good capillary refill in nail beds, no clubbing, cyanosis, or edema.

PERIPHERAL PULSES: 2+ dorsalis pedis, 2+ posterior tibial, 2+ radial.

NEUROLOGIC: nonfocal, alert and oriented.

Critical Thinking:

1) What are the major concerns in this case?
2) What is your plan for Ali?
3) What teaching is appropriate at this time?

Ethan

HPI: Ethan is a 35-year-old Latino diabetic male who presents for a FU visit and medication refills. Today, he denies health complaints. He denies signs or symptoms of hypoglycemia. He saw an eye doctor last week because he got something in his eyes at work. He has a FU appointment next week. He rarely checks his BG. One week ago, his BG was 185 three hours after a meal. Ethan eats five tortillas daily along with bread, meat, and soda. He eats minimal fruit and vegetables. Ethan denies HA, chest pain, dyspnea, or GI/GU problems. He has occasional numbness/tingling in his feet after walking a lot.

Medications:

Metformin HCL 1000 mg 1 tablet with a meal twice a day.
Lisinopril 10 mg 1 tablet once a day.
Simvastatin 20 mg 1 tablet once a day.

Glipizide 10 mg 1 tablet 30 minutes before breakfast and dinner, twice a day.

Medical/Surgical History:

Diabetes mellitus type 2.
Hyperlipidemia.
Hypertension.

FMH:

Both parents are deceased, related to complications of diabetes. His father also had hypertension.
Six sisters; one son: alive and well.

SH:

Smokes approximately five cigarettes/day for 15 years. Drinks 10 or more alcoholic drinks (usually beer) daily on most days.
Living with family. Single. Works 25–30 hours/week as an auto mechanic.

Allergies: NKDA.

ROS:

See HPI.

Vital Signs:

Ht 65 in, Wt 173 lbs, BP 124/76 mmHg, HR 86/min, RR 16/min, Temp 97.8 F.

General Examination:

GENERAL APPEARANCE: alert, well hydrated, in no distress.
EYES: sclera are pink, BL pupils equal, round, reactive to light and accommodation, extraocular movement intact.
ORAL CAVITY: mucosa moist, good dentition, missing one tooth lower left.
NECK/THYROID: no cervical lymphadenopathy, no thyroid nodules, no thyromegaly.

SKIN: warm and dry, no suspicious lesions, no rashes.

HEART: S1, S2 normal, regular rate and rhythm, no murmurs, rubs, gallops, no clicks.

LUNGS: clear to auscultation bilaterally.

EXTREMITIES: good capillary refill in nail beds, no clubbing, cyanosis, or edema.

PERIPHERAL PULSES: 2+ dorsalis pedis, 2+ posterior tibial, 2+ radial.

NEUROLOGIC: nonfocal, alert and oriented, cerebellar function normal, cognitive exam grossly normal, cooperative with exam, no rigidity, no tremor.

PSYCH: alert, oriented, cognitive function intact, cooperative with exam, good eye contact, judgment and insight good, speech clear, thought content without suicidal ideation, delusions.

FOOT EXAM: sensory testing performed: sensations diminished. Sensory and motor testing performed: strength normal. Pedal pulse taking performed: 2+. Visual inspection: normal.

Critical Thinking:

1) What are the major concerns in this case?
2) What is your plan for Ethan?
3) What teaching is appropriate at this time?

Juan

HPI: Juan is a 19-year-old Latino male who went to the hospital emergency department (ED) with left flank pain. He was diagnosed with kidney stones and was referred to urology. He said he could not afford to see the urologist but was given Percocet 5/325 and ibuprofen 600 mg. His friend told him about this clinic, so he made an appointment. He presents today as a new patient with left flank pain and a diagnosis of kidney stones. He does not have any ED discharge paperwork.

Medications:

Amoxicillin of unknown dose (obtained from Latin store).
Percocet 5/325 mg.
Ibuprofen 600 mg.

Medical/Surgical History:

Kidney stones.

FMH:

Sister with history of kidney stones.

SH:

Works as a landscaper. Uses minimal alcohol. Denies tobacco or recreational drug use.

Allergies: NKDA.

ROS:

HEENT: Juan has never had vision or dental exams. Denies headaches, visual changes, nasal congestion, sinus pain, sore throat.

Cardiovascular/respiratory: denies chest pain, difficulty breathing, or pain with breathing.

GI/GU: reports occasional constipation. Juan drinks 2 liters of water daily. He eats very little fruit or vegetables. He eats mostly fried and fast food. Juan denies blood in his stool. Juan reports a previous episode of a kidney stone last year that resolved on its own. He had pain but did not go to the hospital. Today, he reports severe left flank pain 7–8/10 and gross hematuria. He has difficulty sleeping due to the pain. Juan took Amoxicillin of unknown dose that he got from the Latin store down the street. He took Amoxicillin once a day for three days prior to this visit. He denies fever, chills, nausea, vomiting, or diarrhea.

Musculoskeletal: reports frequent LBP due to bending over a lot at work. He denies heavy lifting.

Skin: denies dry skin, open lesions, suspicious lesions.

Psychiatric: reports anxiety due to constant pain.

Vital Signs:

Ht 65 in, Wt 150 lbs, BP 120/80 mmHg, HR 64/min, RR 16/min.

General Examination:

GENERAL APPEARANCE: alert and oriented ×4, well hydrated, NAD, stoic.
EYES: pupils equal, round, reactive to light and accommodation.
NECK: no lymphadenopathy.
SKIN: warm and dry.
HEART: S1, S2 normal, regular rate and rhythm, no murmurs, rubs, gallops, no clicks.
LUNGS: clear to auscultation bilaterally.
ABDOMEN: +CVAT left side, +BS, soft, NT, no HSM, no rebound, no guarding or rigidity.
EXTREMITIES: good capillary refill in nail beds, no clubbing, cyanosis, or edema.
PERIPHERAL PULSES: 2+ radial.
NEUROLOGIC: nonfocal, alert and oriented.

Critical Thinking:

1) What are the major concerns in this case?
2) What is your plan for Juan?
3) What patient teaching is appropriate at this time?

Margarita

HPI: 57-year-old female, Margarita, reports pain in the right side of her hip. She fell in her house outside of the bathroom. Five days ago, she had a bad headache but went to work the next day. She came home from work, took a shower, and went to sleep and awoke the next day with a headache. On getting OOB yesterday, the patient went to the bathroom. As she was leaving the bathroom, she suddenly fell backward on the floor. She hit the back of her head but denies loss of consciousness. She felt cold and sweaty. Her sister took her blood pressure immediately following the fall, but it was "unreadable with error messages." Her sister then took her blood sugar, which was 105. Margarita says she went to bed to lie down. She then felt pain in her right hip and lower back and her headache became worse. She describes right hip/back pain as >10/10, but headache is minimal today. She reports pain with walking. She has been using Inflamma-X (turmeric, tart cherry, protease enzymes, Boswellia) and has used cupping to relieve the pain. Neither remedy has provided much relief. The patient works caring for an elderly person. She denies vision or memory/mentation changes. Margarita cannot recall her last medical visit or when she last had any blood work.

Medications:

Trazodone 50 mg tablets, 1 tablet once a day as needed for sleep.
Sumatriptan succinate 50 mg tablet.
[Pt has not taken these medicines for a long time.]

Medical/Surgical History:

Partial hysterectomy.
Cholecystectomy.
Headaches.

FMH:

Father: deceased, hypertension, kidney disease, anemia, depression, arthritis, hypothyroidism, hyperlipidemia, diagnosed with stroke.
Mother: deceased, died from meningitis.
Ages unknown.

SH:

Denies use of tobacco, alcohol, or recreational drugs.
Living with family, single, works full time.

OB/GYN History:

No pregnancies.
Postmenopausal.
Never had a mammogram or Pap smear.

Allergies:
Penicillin: rash—allergy.

Vital Signs:

Ht 65 in, Wt 170 lbs, BP 120/74 mmHg, HR 86/min, RR 16/min, Temp 97.8 F.

General Examination:

GENERAL APPEARANCE: obese, moves slowly and with visible pain, alert and oriented ×3.

HEAD: normocephalic, atraumatic, no scalp lesions/swelling.

EYES: pupils equal, round, reactive to light and accommodation, extraocular movement intact.

SKIN: warm and dry. Cupping scars are noted on chest and abdomen.

HEART: S1, S2 normal, regular rate and rhythm, no murmurs, rubs, gallops, no clicks.

LUNGS: clear to auscultation bilaterally.

ABDOMEN: bowel sounds present, soft, nontender, nondistended, no hepatosplenomegaly.

BACK: pain on ROM: rotation and extension. No pain on flexion.

MUSCULOSKELETAL: pain on palpation of right hip and LB. Negative SLR BL. Pt has right inguinal pain on flexion and extension of right hip. Able to walk with minimal pain, if she takes small steps.

EXTREMITIES: good capillary refill in nail beds, no clubbing, cyanosis, or edema.

PERIPHERAL PULSES: 2+ dorsalis pedis, 2+ posterior tibial, 2+ radial.

NEUROLOGIC: nonfocal, alert and oriented.

Patient was given Toradol 60 mg IM in the clinic with moderate relief after 30 minutes.

Critical Thinking:

1) What are the major concerns in this case?
2) What is your plan for Margarita?
3) What patient teaching is appropriate at this time?

Paula

HPI: Paula is a 60-year-old Latina female who presents with report of a productive cough with yellowish sputum for one month. She also reports headache, "fever" (she has not taken her temperature), and dyspnea for 15 days.

She is taking Tylenol, Mucinex, and a tea that contains garlic and onion. She stopped all of her other medications. She didn't think she should take them because she didn't feel well. She denies nausea, vomiting, diarrhea.

Medications:

Tylenol 1 tablet prn headache.
Mucinex 600 mg Extended Release 1 tablet as needed every 12 hours.
She is not taking the following previous prescriptions:
Atorvastatin 20 1 tablet daily in evening.
Omeprazole 20 mg delayed release 1 capsule 30 minutes before morning meal.
Metformin 500 mg 1 tablet twice a day.
Lisinopril 20 mg tablets, 1 tablet once a day.
Hydrochlorothiazide 25 mg 1 tablet once a day.
MiraLAX powder as directed every night.
Metamucil 48.57% powder as directed every morning.
Vitamin D 2000 unit tablet, 1 tablet once a day.

Medical/Surgical History:

Acid reflux.
Hyperlipidemia.
Hypertension.
Constipation.
Prediabetes.
Vitamin D deficiency.

FMH:

Mother: deceased, cause of death: alcoholism, depression.
Father: deceased, HTN, hyperlipidemia.
Eight siblings: two brothers are deceased d/t unknown causes, one sister has DMT2, the remainder have HTN and hyperlipidemia.

OB/GYN History:

Seven pregnancies, seven NSVD, live children.
Currently sexually active.
Last Pap smear: unsure of date or result.
Last mammogram: two years ago, negative.

Postmenopausal since age 45.
Sexually transmitted diseases: none.

Allergies:
None.

ROS:

HEENT: admits to HA × 15 days. Reports BL facial pain and forehead pain. Denies problems with vision or hearing or vertigo. Denies nasal congestion or sore throat.
Cardiovascular/respiratory: admits to cough with sputum production. Denies chest pain, dizziness, hemoptysis, pain with inspiration, shortness of breath at rest or with exertion.
GI/GU: denies abdominal pain. Denies blood in stool or urine, change in bowel habits, difficulty urinating.

Vital Signs:

Ht 60 in, Wt 172 lbs, BP 140/66 mmHg, HR 80/min, RR 16/min, Temp 97.6 F.

General Examination:

GENERAL APPEARANCE: alert, well hydrated, in no distress.
HEAD: normocephalic, atraumatic.
EYES: pupils equal, round, reactive to light and accommodation, extraocular movement intact.
EARS: tympanic membrane intact.
NOSE: +BL maxillary and ethmoid sinus TTP, clear discharge, nares patent.
ORAL CAVITY: mucosa moist.
THROAT: no erythema, no exudate, pharynx normal.
NECK/THYROID: no cervical lymphadenopathy.
SKIN: warm and dry.
HEART: S1, S2 normal, regular rate and rhythm, no murmurs, rubs, gallops, no clicks.
LUNGS: clear to auscultation bilaterally, clear anteriorly and posteriorly.
EXTREMITIES: good capillary refill in nail beds, no clubbing, cyanosis, or edema.
PERIPHERAL PULSES: 2+ dorsalis pedis, 2+ posterior tibial, 2+ radial.
NEUROLOGIC: nonfocal, alert and oriented.

Critical Thinking:

1) What are the major concerns in this case?
2) What is your plan for Paula?
3) What teaching is appropriate at this time?

Rosa

HPI: Rosa, a 61-year-old Latina female, presents to the clinic for review of blood work results. She reports pain and swelling in the third digit of her right hand. She works cleaning washing machines at a laundromat. She develops blisters on her fingers despite wearing rubber gloves. The blister on the third digit right hand became swollen and painful, so she popped it with a needle and pushed out yellow pus. She then soaked it in salt water followed by "water with herbs." She has not been working for one week because the finger is now very painful. She purchased Amoxicillin and ibuprofen at the local Latin store. She has been taking 500 mg of Amoxicillin three times a day for eight days. She takes ibuprofen (unknown dose) twice a day with minimal relief. Rosa is out of her blood pressure and cholesterol medications.

Medications:

Amoxicillin 500 mg three times a day.
Ibuprofen twice a day.
Lisinopril 20 mg daily.
Simvastatin 20 mg daily.

Medical/Surgical History:

Hypertension.
Hyperlipidemia.

FMH:

Mother and father died in patient's home country of unknown causes.
 They were each in their 60s.

SH:

Pt does not use tobacco, alcohol, or recreational drugs.

Allergies: NKDA.

ROS:

HEENT: denies headaches or changes in vision; denies epistaxis.
Cardiovascular/respiratory: denies chest pain, dyspnea, hemoptysis.
Musculoskeletal: see HPI.
Neurological: denies headache, dizziness.

Vital Signs:

Ht 62 in, Wt 185 lbs, BP 150/90 mmHg, HR 76/min, RR 16/min.

General Examination:

GENERAL: alert and oriented ×4, NAD.
EYES: PERRLA.
SKIN: warm and dry.
HEART: NSR, Regular rate and rhythm S1, S2, no murmurs, clicks, gallops, rubs.
RESPIRATORY: CTA BL.
MUSCULOSKELETAL: the third digit of the right hand is erythematous; there is signficant swelling of the entire finger and a nodule in the DIP joint. The patient is unable to fully flex or extend the finger without pain.
NEUROLOGICAL: cooperative, cognition grossly intact, Romberg negative, DTRs +2 UEs and LEs, no rigidity or tremor.
Patient's recent lab work: UA, CBC, TSH, CMP, FIT were all WNL.

Critical Thinking:

1) What are the major concerns in this case?
2) What is your plan for Rosa?
3) What teaching is appropriate at this time?

Santiago

HPI: Santiago is a 53-year-old Latino male who presents as a new patient with DMT2. He has not had been taking any medicine, other than occasional metformin, for three years. Someone sends him metformin from his country. He had been taking 500 mg in the morning for six months but stopped six months ago. He was diagnosed with DM 10 years ago. He states he is very tired and has lost 30 pounds since arriving in the United States three years ago.

Medications:

None.

Medical/Surgical History:

DMT2.

FMH:

Mother: deceased age 70 of unknown cancer.
Father: deceased age 60 of DM.

SH:

Denies use of tobacco, alcohol, or recreational drugs.
Living alone, single, works part time in a restaurant kitchen.
Not currently sexually active.
Sexually transmitted diseases: none.

ROS:

General/constitutional: tires easily when walking. Denies change in appetite. Denies sleep disturbance. Denies weight gain or loss.
HEENT: reports dental pain and missing teeth. Denies headaches, problems with vision, difficulty swallowing or hearing, nasal congestion, sore throat.
Endocrine: denies cold or heat intolerance, difficulty sleeping.
Cardiovascular/respiratory: denies chest pain, dizziness, palpitations, edema, pain with inspiration, shortness of breath at rest or with exertion.
GI/GU: denies abdominal pain, blood in urine or stool, constipation, nausea, vomiting, diarrhea, difficulty urinating.
Psychiatric: denies anxiety.
Musculoskeletal: reports burning sensation in the skin of his lower back, waist, and left leg × six months. He works with frozen products in a Latin supermarket and lifts heavy things. He was told he had neuropathy.
Neurologic: denies tingling/numbness.

Vital Signs:

Ht 65 in, Wt 150 lbs, BP 130/96mmHg, HR 72/min, RR 16/min, Temp 98.3 F.

General Examination:

GENERAL APPEARANCE: alert, well hydrated, in no distress.

HEAD: normocephalic, atraumatic.

EYES: pupils equal, round, reactive to light and accommodation, extraocular movement intact.

EARS: tympanic membrane intact, clear.

ORAL CAVITY: poor dentition, mucosa moist. No visible abscesses, ulcers, lesions, inflammation, or swelling.

THROAT: no erythema, no exudate, pharynx normal.

NECK/THYROID: carotid pulse normal, no carotid bruit, neck supple, full range of motion, no cervical lymphadenopathy, no jugular venous distention, no thyroid nodules, no thyromegaly, thyroid nontender.

SKIN: warm and dry, no rashes, no acanthosis.

HEART: regularly irregular HR/radial pulse, S1, S2, no murmurs, rubs, gallops, no clicks.

LUNGS: clear to auscultation bilaterally.

ABDOMEN: bowel sounds present, soft, nontender, nondistended, no hepatosplenomegaly, no guarding or rigidity.

BACK: no costovertebral angle tenderness, normal exam of spine, spine nontender to palpation.

MUSCULOSKELETAL: cervical spine normal, full range of motion of the hip, lumbosacral spine normal, no swelling or deformity.

EXTREMITIES: good capillary refill in nail beds, no clubbing, cyanosis, or edema.

PERIPHERAL PULSES: 2+ dorsalis pedis, 2+ posterior tibial, 2+ radial.

NEUROLOGIC: nonfocal, alert and oriented, cognitive exam grossly normal, cooperative with exam, cranial nerves 2–12 grossly intact, deep tendon reflexes 2+ symmetrical, gait normal, motor strength normal upper and lower extremities, no rigidity, no tremor.

PODIATRIC: sensation is grossly intact to light touch, no calluses or lesions.

PSYCH: alert, oriented, cognitive function intact, cooperative with exam, good eye contact, judgment and insight good, speech clear, thought content without suicidal ideation, delusions.

Critical Thinking:

1) What are the major concerns in this case?
2) What is your plan of treatment?
3) What should be included in patient teaching for Santiago?

3

Food or Housing Issues

Carmen

HPI: Carmen, a 60-year-old Latina female, reports that three weeks ago, she felt like "my heart was accelerated, but now I feel fine." The symptoms occurred while she was lying down preparing to go to sleep. She denies association with anxiety. She did not check her blood pressure. Carmen says she feels "weak" because she is not eating meat, partly due to the cost and partly due to concern about her cholesterol. She cannot afford fruit.

Medications:

Vitamin D3 2000 unit 1 capsule once a day.
Levothyroxine sodium 75 mcg 1 tablet in the morning on an empty stomach once a day.
Atorvastatin calcium 40 mg 1 tablet once a day.
Omega 3 1000 mg 1 capsule once a day.

Medical/Surgical History:

Hyperlipidemia.
Epigastric pain.

Caring for the Displaced and Uninsured: Clinical Case Studies in Nursing & Healthcare, First Edition. Leslie Neal-Boylan.
© 2023 John Wiley & Sons Ltd. Published 2023 by John Wiley & Sons Ltd.

FMH:

Father: deceased, alcohol abuse.
Mother: alive, arthritis, hypertension.
Siblings and children are healthy.

SH:

Denies use of tobacco, alcohol, or recreational drugs. Lives alone.

OB/GYN History:

No pregnancies.
Not currently sexually active.
Last Pap smear: two years ago, negative.
Last mammogram: two years ago, bi-rad 1.
Postmenopausal × 10 years.
Birth control: none.

Allergies: Azithromycin—rash.

ROS:

Cardiovascular/respiratory: denies chest pain, pain with inspiration, shortness of breath at rest or with exertion, dizziness, edema.
GI/GU: denies abdominal pain, blood in stool or urine, change in bowel habits, or difficulty urinating.
Skin: denies skin concerns.
Neurologic: admits loss of strength. Denies memory loss, dizziness, tingling/numbness.

Vital Signs:

Ht 54 in, Wt 90 lbs, BP 124/70 mmHg, HR 70/min, RR 14/min, Temp 98.2 F.

General Examination:

GENERAL APPEARANCE: alert, well hydrated, in no distress.
EYES: pupils equal, round, reactive to light and accommodation.

HEART: S1, S2 normal, regular rate and rhythm, no murmurs, rubs, gallops, no clicks.

LUNGS: clear to auscultation bilaterally.

EXTREMITIES: good capillary refill in nail beds, no clubbing, cyanosis, or edema. PERIPHERAL PULSES: 2+ dorsalis pedis, 2+ posterior tibial, 2+ radial.

NEUROLOGIC: alert and oriented, cognitive exam grossly normal, cooperative with exam.

Critical Thinking:

1) What are the major concerns in this case?
2) What is your plan for Carmen?
3) What teaching is appropriate at this time?

Luciana

HPI: Luciana, a 35-year-old Latina female, returns to the clinic after a two-year absence. She arrived one hour late to this appointment, saying she took several buses and walked an additional two miles. She said she was "pushed" out of an apartment building before she came here because she was trying to get a place to live and didn't have the necessary paperwork. She reports that the apartment manager refused to speak with her because she only speaks Spanish. She presents today because she has had pain in her left leg since varicose vein surgery six months ago. Burning pain starts in the left knee and moves up to the groin and thigh. She denies a history of sciatica. She reports she feels overwhelmed.

Medications:

Tylenol 650 mg every 4 hours prn pain.

Medical/Surgical History:

Colon cancer ten years ago, treated with chemotherapy and radiation.
Varicose veins, surgery six months ago.
Gestational diabetes.

FMH:

Father: deceased, murdered.
Mother: deceased, diabetes mellitus.

Allergies: Amoxicillin—itching.

SH:

Denies use of tobacco, alcohol, or recreational drugs.

ROS:

HEENT: denies headaches or changes in vision; denies epistaxis or dental problems.

Cardiovascular/respiratory: denies chest pain, dizziness, palpitations, fluid accumulation in the legs, dyspnea, hemoptysis, shortness of breath at rest or with exertion.

GI/GU: denies abdominal pain, blood in stool or urine, change in bowel habits.

Skin: denies problems with hair, skin, nails.

Musculoskeletal: pain in left leg since varicose vein surgery. See HPI.

Neurologic: denies balance difficulty, gait abnormality.

Psychiatric: reports feeling "overwhelmed." Denies depression, SI, or thoughts of harming herself or others.

Neurological: denies numbness/tingling, tremors.

Vital Signs:

Ht 62 in, Wt 205 lbs, BP 135/82 mmHg, HR 106/min, RR 16/min, Temp 96.7 F.

General Examination:

GENERAL APPEARANCE: overweight, unkempt, alert, well hydrated, in no distress.

EYES: pupils equal, round, reactive to light and accommodation.

SKIN: mildly diaphoretic (it is a hot day today; Pt walked partway to come here).

HEART: S1, S2 normal, regular rate and rhythm, no murmurs, rubs, gallops, no clicks.

LUNGS: clear to auscultation bilaterally.

MUSCULOSKELETAL: left leg above knee is covered with large Band-Aid. Skin reveals two healed puncture wounds, no apparent swelling. No signs of possible DVT, no swelling, warmth, redness, no streaking. PPP BL.

Addendum: clinician notes that Luciana walks slowly, limping into waiting room, and requests help to walk to her car.

PSYCH: a bit scattered, questionable historian.

Luciana is told to take Tylenol or ibuprofen with food for leg pain and apply warm compresses to the area of the leg that hurts. She is told to go to the ED if pain becomes worse or she develops redness, warmth, or swelling. The clinic pays for a taxi to take Luciana home.

Luciana follows up in four weeks:

HPI: she presents after canceling two appointments. She wants a referral to neurology and a note saying the apartment manager caused her back and leg pain. Luciana reiterates her story saying she had complained to the manager about discrimination. Then the manager pushed her to get her to leave the office. She contacted the police, who told her she needs a note from her doctor to file a complaint.

Vital Signs:

BP 130/76 mmHg, HR 86/min, RR 16/min, Temp 97.5 F.

General Examination:

GENERAL APPEARANCE: obese, alert, well hydrated. Luciana is clearly agitated about her living situation. She interrupts frequently to repeat her story.

NEUROLOGIC: alert and oriented, Luciana does not want to leave the exam room or clinic. She is very agitated and wants a note right now. Her gait is normal today, although during the last visit, she could barely move; no tremor, no rigidity noted today.

PSYCH: alert, oriented, questionable cognitive function, good eye contact, speech clear, thought content without suicidal ideation, delusions. She is insisting on x-rays to prove injury.

Critical Thinking:

1) What are the major concerns in this case?
2) What is your plan for Luciana?
3) What teaching is appropriate at this time?

Michelle

HPI: Michelle, 38-year-old African female, is a new patient seeking primary care. She comes from a homeless shelter. She reports pelvic pain, fatigue, and heavy menstrual bleeding. She was previously informed she has a uterine prolapse requiring surgery. She is living in a shelter with her two young children because her husband is abusive to her. She has a restraining order and is connected to adult and child protective services. Michelle denies that her husband has hurt the children. She says she was told by the shelter to come to the clinic. She has had two miscarriages. She thinks she had some uterine and bladder repair at that time. She does not want to recuperate from surgery in a shelter and has nowhere to keep her children during or after surgery. She says her husband has frightened her friends away, so she is alone.

Medications:

None.

Medical/Surgical History:

Two miscarriages.
Possible bladder repair.

FMH:

Both parents are deceased. Children are alive and well.

Allergies: NKDA

SH:

Denies use of tobacco, alcohol, or recreational drugs. Unemployed. See HPI.

OB/GYN History:

Four pregnancies: two NSVD, two miscarriages.
Periods: irregular, sometimes skips a month. Periods last three or four
    days, not heavy, minimal cramping.

Not currently sexually active.

Last Pap smear: three years ago, normal.

Date of last period: one month ago, does not recall date.

Sexually transmitted diseases: none.

Birth control: none.

Vital Signs:

Ht 72 in, Wt 143 lbs, BP 109/78 mmHg, HR 90/min, RR 14/min, Temp 97.6 F.

General Examination:

GENERAL APPEARANCE: very tearful, alert and oriented ×3, cooperative, visibly upset.

HEAD: normocephalic, atraumatic.

EYES: pupils equal, round, reactive to light and accommodation, extraocular movement intact.

SKIN: warm and dry.

HEART: S1, S2 normal, regular rate and rhythm, no murmurs, rubs, gallops, no clicks.

LUNGS: clear to auscultation bilaterally.

PERIPHERAL PULSES: 2+ radial.

NEUROLOGIC: nonfocal, alert and oriented.

PSYCH: crying, upset, alert, oriented, cognitive function intact, cooperative with exam, good eye contact, judgment and insight good, speech clear, thought content without suicidal ideation, delusions.

Critical Thinking:

1) What are the major concerns in this case?
2) What is your plan for Michelle?
3) What teaching is appropriate at this time?

Paul

HPI: Paul, age 54, is a male diabetic patient returning to the clinic after two years. He says he has been out of medicine for approximately six months. Medicine is sent to him from his home country. Today, he would like a follow-up. He reports he had severe RUQ abdominal pain that "mostly went away" after he stopped drinking eight cups of coffee per day. Eating helps to resolve mild pain after about 20 minutes. He denies that pain is associated with any food. It is most common when he is hungry. Paul admits to constipation, having one hard stool every two to three days without bleeding. He denies nausea, diarrhea, vomiting, blood in the stool. Paul describes his typical diet: fish, fast food chicken, lemonade. He does not drink soda. He does not eat fruit or vegetables, except an occasional apple. He does not drink water. He says he sometimes drinks Gatorade. He does not check his blood sugar. He denies signs or symptoms of hypoglycemia. Typical diet includes rice, beans, pasta, and tortillas.

Medications:

He is not taking Novolin 70/30, metformin, glipizide, or rosuvastatin prescribed during last visit because he ran out of medicine.

Medical/Surgical History:

Type 2 diabetes mellitus.
Hyperlipidemia.
Appendectomy in home country, date unknown.

FMH:

Mother is deceased, unknown age at death, unknown cause of death.
Father: alive, age 62, DM, heart disease.
Spouse and children are in Pt's home country.

SH:

Smoker: one pack per day for 22 years. Occasionally (once or twice per week), he smokes marijuana. He drinks four 16-oz beers on a weekend day. He lives alone. Pt reports the local priest wakes him to walk daily. Paul used to sleep on the floor of a basement of the house of one of the church's parishioners. He sends money back to his home country. The priest paid for a bed because the patient developed low back pain when sleeping on the floor. He works full time making product deliveries.

ROS:

HEENT: denies headaches, problems with vision. The patient has never been to an eye doctor. He denies dental pain. He has never seen a dentist. He was hit in the mouth several years ago in his home country. He would like to get his teeth fixed. Cardiovascular/respiratory: Pt admits to fluid accumulation in legs. Denies chest pain, dizziness, or palpitations. Denies cough, hemoptysis, pain with inspiration, shortness of breath at rest or with exertion. GI/GU: admits to abdominal pain, constipation, heartburn. Denies blood in the stool or urine, diarrhea, nausea, vomiting. Admits to urinary frequency. Denies difficulty urinating, current sexual activity. Skin: reports intermittent rash on arms and legs. Applies bleach to skin to decrease itching. Neurologic: denies tingling/numbness. Psychiatric: admits to work stress and worry about family in home country. Denies anxiety, depressed mood.

Vital Signs:

Ht 66.5 in, Wt 250 lbs, BP 140/90 mmHg, HR 80/min, RR 16/min, Temp 98.4 F, FBG 275.

General Examination:

GENERAL APPEARANCE: obese, alert, well hydrated, in no distress.
HEAD: normocephalic, atraumatic.
EYES: pupils equal, round, reactive to light and accommodation, extraocular movement intact.
NECK/THYROID: no cervical lymphadenopathy, no jugular venous distention, no thyroid nodules, no thyromegaly, thyroid nontender.
SKIN: warm and dry.
HEART: S1, S2 normal, regular rate and rhythm, no murmurs, rubs, gallops, no clicks.
LUNGS: clear anteriorly and posteriorly.
ABDOMEN: obese, bowel sounds present, soft, nontender, nondistended, no hepatosplenomegaly, no guarding or rigidity.
BACK: normal exam of spine, spine nontender to palpation, no costovertebral angle tenderness.
MUSCULOSKELETAL: cervical spine normal, full range of motion of the hip, lumbosacral spine normal, no swelling or deformity.
EXTREMITIES: good capillary refill in nail beds, no clubbing, cyanosis, or edema.

PERIPHERAL PULSES: 2+ dorsalis pedis, 2+ posterior tibial, 2+ radial.
NEUROLOGIC: alert and oriented, cerebellar function normal, cognitive exam grossly normal, cooperative with exam, cranial nerves II–XII grossly intact, deep tendon reflexes 2+ symmetrical, gait normal, motor strength normal upper and lower extremities.
PODIATRIC: poor sensation on testing with monofilament, bilaterally right is worse than left, poor vibratory sensation in BL feet.
PSYCH: alert, oriented, cognitive function intact, cooperative with exam, good eye contact, judgment and insight good, speech clear, thought content without suicidal ideation, delusions.

Results of Blood Work:

LDL—101.
HA1c 8.4%.

Critical Thinking:

1) What are the major concerns in this case?
2) What is your plan for Paul?
3) What teaching is appropriate at this time?

4

Financial Issues

Glenda

HPI: 65-year-old female Glenda presents for lab results and refills of her medications. Glenda was last here one year ago. She states she has asthma attacks every night. A friend gave her Advair, which she takes occasionally and only in the evening because it is expensive. She uses an "albuterol inhaler" every night and sometimes alternates it with Ventolin. She does not have a nebulizer. Glenda also reports frequent abdominal pain that is relieved by Tums. She only takes glipizide for DM because metformin upsets her stomach. She also reports pain in her right knee and in her left hip, radiating from left mid-back to her left leg and ankle. She works part time as a home health aide. Glenda reports going to the ED during one asthma episode. She felt like she was treated differently once staff found out she does not have insurance.

Medications:

Montelukast 100 mg.
Gabapentin 10 mg.
Glipizide 5 mg.
Ventolin.
Albuterol inhaler.

Caring for the Displaced and Uninsured: Clinical Case Studies in Nursing & Healthcare, First Edition. Leslie Neal-Boylan.

Medical/Surgical History:

Diabetes mellitus type 2.
Osteoarthritis.
Asthma since age 15 years.

Allergies: Metformin HCL—rash, dizziness, GI distress.

FMH:

Father: deceased, family history unknown.
Mother: deceased, family history unknown.
Paternal grandmother: deceased, diagnosed with diabetes.

SH:

Denies use of tobacco, alcohol, recreational drugs.

ROS:

HEENT: Glenda reports intermittent headaches when she feels stressed. She uses reading glasses; she had prescription glasses for distance vision, but they broke, and she doesn't have the money to replace them. She reports multiple dental "cavities" that cause pain. She has never been to a dentist or had an eye exam.

Cardiovascular/respiratory: denies chest pain at rest or with exertion. She denies dizziness or palpitations. She occasionally has fluid accumulation in her legs. She reports feeling short of breath at night. She uses several pillows to sleep comfortably. She was never a smoker, but her husband was a heavy smoker. Glenda had a normal CXR sometime previously. She denies chest, cough, hemoptysis, pain with inspiration.

GI/GU: she uses Ex-Lax a few times/week. She denies abdominal pain, blood in stool, or constipation. She reports stress incontinence and urinary urgency. Nocturia ×2. She drinks "a lot" of water throughout the day and tea at night. She denies blood in the urine and difficulty urinating.

Musculoskeletal: reports left hip pain and right knee pain. She refuses x-rays.

Neurologic: she reports tingling/numbness from mid-back to left hip and leg.

Psychiatric: reports anxiety; she worries about her health. She denies depression.

Vital Signs:

Ht 63 in, Wt 240 lbs, BP 144/90 mmHg, HR 76/min, RR 16/min, Temp 97.9 F.

General Examination:

GENERAL APPEARANCE: obese, alert, well hydrated, in no distress, well developed, well nourished.

HEAD: normocephalic, atraumatic.

EYES: pupils equal, round, reactive to light and accommodation, extraocular movement intact, fundus normal.

NECK/THYROID: no cervical lymphadenopathy, no jugular venous distention, no carotid bruit, carotid pulse normal, neck supple, full range of motion, no thyromegaly.

SKIN: no suspicious lesions, normal hair distribution, warm and dry.

HEART: S1, S2 normal, regular rate and rhythm, no murmurs, rubs, gallops, no clicks.

LUNGS: wheezes throughout lungs bilaterally.

ABDOMEN: bowel sounds present, soft, nontender, nondistended, no hepatosplenomegaly.

MUSCULOSKELETAL: no swelling or deformity negative SLR bilaterally, Pain in left hip with ROM, no pain with ROM of knees, Strength in UEs and LEs is 5/5.

EXTREMITIES: good capillary refill in nail beds, no clubbing, cyanosis, or edema.

PERIPHERAL PULSES: 2+ dorsalis pedis, 2+ posterior tibial, 2+ posterior tibial.

NEUROLOGIC: alert and oriented, cerebellar function normal, cognitive exam grossly normal, cooperative with exam, cranial nerves II–XII grossly intact, deep tendon reflexes 2+ symmetrical, gait normal, motor strength normal upper and lower extremities.

PSYCH: alert, oriented, cognitive function intact, cooperative with exam, good eye contact, judgment and insight good, speech clear, thought content without suicidal ideation, delusions.

Pulse ox 98%.

Critical Thinking:

1) What are the major concerns in this case?
2) What is your plan for Glenda?
3) What teaching is appropriate at this time?

Guillermo

HPI: Guillermo is a 30-year-old Latino male presenting as a new patient. He reports abdominal pain in the morning and has been feeling tired all of the time for three years. He was positive for *H. Pylori* in his home country but could not continue treatment due to the expense. He reports discomfort in his abdomen, anal itching, headache, dizziness, nausea without vomiting or diarrhea, and knee pain. His last medical visit was six months ago in his home country. He was given a special diet, but he could not finish it. He says he cannot work because he has not felt well. He does not take any medicine. His symptoms are worse with fried and spicy foods. Eating fruit helps. He does not drink soda or alcohol. He has had constipation but denies blood in the stool or urine. He reports frequency of urination but no dysuria.

Medications:

None.

Medical/Surgical History:

Positive *H. Pylori*.

FMH:

Parents and one sibling are alive and well. He does not have a partner or children.

SH:

Denies use of tobacco, alcohol, or recreational drugs. Living with sister; he is single, unemployed.

Vital Signs:

Ht 65 in, Wt 148 lbs 8 oz, BP 134/72 mmHg, HR 62/min, RR 16/min, Temp 98.6 F.

General Examination:

GENERAL APPEARANCE: alert, well hydrated, in no distress.
HEAD: normocephalic, atraumatic.

EYES: pupils equal, round, reactive to light and accommodation, extraocular movement intact.

NECK/THYROID: no cervical lymphadenopathy, no thyroid nodules, no thyromegaly.

SKIN: warm and dry.

HEART: S1, S2 normal, regular rate and rhythm, no murmurs, rubs, gallops, no clicks. LUNGS: clear to auscultation bilaterally.

ABDOMEN: bowel sounds present, RUQ TTP, otherwise NT, no hepatosplenomegaly, no guarding or rigidity, negative Murphy's sign.

BACK: no costovertebral angle tenderness.

RECTAL: no hemorrhoids, fissures, bleeding, melena. Guaiac is negative.

EXTREMITIES: good capillary refill in nail beds, no clubbing, cyanosis, or edema.

PERIPHERAL PULSES: 2+ dorsalis pedis, 2+ posterior tibial, 2+ radial.

NEUROLOGIC: nonfocal, alert and oriented. Steady gait. Romberg is negative.

PSYCH: alert, oriented, cognitive function intact, cooperative with exam, good eye contact, judgment, and insight good, speech clear, thought content without suicidal ideation, delusions.

Critical Thinking:

1) What are the major concerns in this case?
2) What is your plan for Guillermo?
3) What teaching is appropriate at this time?

Lisette

HPI: Lisette, a 65-year-old female, presents with left foot pain, itching, and swelling for one week. Lisette has not been to the clinic for two years. Her teenaged granddaughter is present to translate. Lisette says she had a similar episode before and was given antibiotics with resolution. She does not recall being bitten by anything but recently saw an insect in her bed. She denies trauma. Lisette went to urgent care for the current problem and was told to go to the ED, but she didn't want to pay the cost. She denies fever or chills. She reports that the left foot becomes very hot; sometimes swelling and redness move up the foot but recede when she elevates the leg. Lisette reports living in another state for one year and being treated there and by phone for DM and hyperlipidemia. She reports she is out of medicine and needs refills. She does not check her BG at home. Lisette says she's supposed to take metformin 500 mg, but her pharmacy didn't have 500 mg so she takes 1000 mg once a day. She also takes glipizide, aspirin, and atorvastatin daily.

Medications:

Aspirin 81 mg delayed release 1 tablet once a day.
Metformin 1000 mg 1 tablet once a day.
Glipizide 5 mg tablet once a day, prebreakfast.
Atorvastatin 40 mg once daily.

Medical/Surgical History:

Diabetes.
Hyperlipidemia.
Hysterectomy—total.

FMH:

Mother: deceased, MI.
Father: deceased, depression.
Five siblings are alive and well, except for one brother with DMT2.
Five children are alive and well.
SH: reports drinking four to five alcoholic drinks (beer or wine) per day. Denies use of tobacco or recreational drugs. Living with family, widowed, unemployed.

OB/GYN History:

Five pregnancies. Five NSVD.
Not currently sexually active.
Last Pap smear: 20 years ago, normal.
Last mammogram: six years ago, bi-rad 2.
Postmenopausal.
Sexually transmitted diseases: none.
Hysterectomy—unknown cause.

Vital Signs:

Ht 62 in, Wt 148 lbs, BP 160/86 mmHg, HR 72/min, RR 16/min, Temp 98.6 F, glucose 150, fasting.

General Examination:

GENERAL APPEARANCE: alert, well hydrated, in no distress.

EYES: pupils equal, round, reactive to light and accommodation.

SKIN: LLE from mid-calf to entire foot is swollen to ~1.5 size of RLE. Skin of anterior calf from mid-calf including anterior ankle is erythematous and warm. Femoral pulses and PP are +2. No streaking. No inguinal lymphadenopathy. No drainage. Pt has pain on palpation and manipulation of LLE.

HEART: S1, S2 normal, regular rate and rhythm, no murmurs, rubs, gallops, no clicks.

LUNGS: clear to auscultation bilaterally.

EXTREMITIES: left calf warm, red, swollen.

PERIPHERAL PULSES: 2+ radial, 2+ femoral, 2+ dorsalis pedis, 2+ posterior tibial.

NEUROLOGIC: nonfocal, alert and oriented.

PSYCH: alert, oriented, cognitive function intact, cooperative with exam, good eye contact, judgment and insight good, speech clear, thought content without suicidal ideation, delusions.

Critical Thinking:

1) What are the major concerns in this case?
2) What is your plan for Lisette?
3) What patient teaching is appropriate at this time?

Lucia

HPI: Lucia, age 35, is a deaf female Latina patient who presents for follow-up of a cholecystectomy two weeks ago. She presents with hearing aids and uses a cell phone and paper and pen to communicate. She reports mild postoperative RUQ pain and is taking Tylenol with relief.

She works in a restaurant kitchen but is not working now. She plans to return to work and is worried about paying medical and other bills while not working and without insurance. Her mother is helping her while she recovers. Lucia saw the surgeon five days ago for FU and was told she is healing well but should not lift heavy things. She reports occasional depression. She denies SI or intention to hurt herself.

Medications:

Tylenol 650 mg every four to six hours prn pain.

Medical/Surgical History:

Hepatitis B, treated.
Hearing loss due to taking gentamicin—wears bilateral hearing aids.
Suicide attempt five years ago.

FMH:

Parents alive with HTN and hyperlipidemia, one brother with DM type 2.

SH:

Drinks six 16-oz beers three times per week. Denies use of tobacco or recreational drugs. Living in mother's basement, single, unemployed.

OB/GYN History:

Never pregnant.
Last period: two weeks ago, normal and regular, last three to four days.
Not sexually active, no birth control.
Last Pap smear: never.

Allergies: NKDA.

ROS:

HEENT: denies headaches, ear pain, nasal congestion, sore throat, or dysphagia.
Cardiovascular/respiratory: denies chest pain, dizziness, palpitations, dyspnea at rest or with exertion, hemoptysis, cough.

GI/GU: admits to abdominal pain, status post–recent surgery. Reports mild pain relieved by Tylenol. Lucia denies bowel or bladder problems, blood in stool or urine, change in bowel or bladder habits, constipation, decreased appetite, nausea, diarrhea, vomiting.

Skin: reports incision is healing and sometimes itching.

Vital Signs:

Ht 65.0 in, Wt 120 lbs, BP 110/64 mmHg, HR 82/min, RR 14/min, Temp 98.0 F.

General Examination:

GENERAL APPEARANCE: alert, well hydrated, in no distress, in no acute distress.

HEAD: normocephalic, atraumatic.

EYES: pupils equal, round, reactive to light and accommodation.

EARS: bilateral hearing aids, speech is unclear.

SKIN: healed abdominal incision. Lucia is wearing a splint around her abdomen.

HEART: S1, S2 normal, regular rate and rhythm, no murmurs, rubs, gallops, no clicks.

LUNGS: clear to auscultation bilaterally.

ABDOMEN: bowel sounds present, healed incision.

NEUROLOGIC: alert and oriented.

PSYCH: alert, oriented, cognitive function intact, cooperative with exam, good eye contact, thought content without suicidal ideation, delusions.

Critical Thinking:

1) What are the major concerns in this case?
2) What is your plan for Lucia?
3) What teaching is appropriate at this time?

5

Work-Related Issues

Karla

HPI: Karla, age 32, presents for FU of pain in her right elbow, numbness and tingling in BL wrists and hands, mid-lower back pain, and BL hip pain for one month. She says she sleeps with her right arm extended on pillow. She works full time cleaning houses. She denies heavy lifting or trauma.

Medications:

Atorvastatin calcium 20 mg 1 tablet once a day.

Medical/Surgical History:

Depression and anxiety.
Hypertension
Hyperlipidemia.

FMH:

Mother is alive. The patient does not know her health status. Her mother
   has never had a medical visit.
Father died age 67 of unknown causes.
Five brothers, six sisters—alive and well.
Patient is single, widowed with three sons, alive and well.

Caring for the Displaced and Uninsured: Clinical Case Studies in Nursing & Healthcare,
First Edition. Leslie Neal-Boylan.
© 2023 John Wiley & Sons Ltd. Published 2023 by John Wiley & Sons Ltd.

SH:

Denies use of tobacco, alcohol, or recreational drugs. Lives with a coworker and coworker's family. Works part time as a painter.

OB/GYN History:

Total pregnancies: four; living children: three NSVD.
Miscarriage: once in home country five years ago.
Periods: sometimes will skip a month or up to two months. For the past two years, periods last for four days with a small amount of blood loss.
LMP—two months ago.
Not currently sexually active.
Last Pap smear date: one year ago, negative.
Sexually transmitted diseases: chlamydia two years ago.
Birth control: none.
Not currently sexually active.

Allergies: NKDA.

Vital Signs:

Ht 61 in, Wt 153 lbs, BP 132/70 mmHg, HR 64/min, RR 16/min, Temp 98.0 F.

General Examination:

GENERAL APPEARANCE: alert and oriented ×3, well developed, well nourished.
EYES: pupils equal, round, reactive to light and accommodation.
SKIN: warm and dry.
HEART: S1, S2 normal, regular rate and rhythm, no murmurs, rubs, gallops, no clicks.
LUNGS: clear to auscultation bilaterally.
ABDOMEN: bowel sounds present, soft, nontender, nondistended, no hepatosplenomegaly, no guarding or rigidity.
MUSCULOSKELETAL: no apparent synovitis, erythema, or nodules of any joint. +MCP squeeze BL. Mild pain on ROM of left thumb, otherwise normal ROM of BL upper extremities, shoulders, arms, wrists, fingers. Negative BL Phalen's test and negative Tinel's test. FROM of trunk, hips, knees without pain. +MTP squeeze BL. No swelling or deformity.

EXTREMITIES: good capillary refill in nail beds, no clubbing, cyanosis, or edema.

PERIPHERAL PULSES: 2+ dorsalis pedis, 2+ dorsalis pedis, 2+ radial.

NEUROLOGIC: nonfocal, alert and oriented, no rigidity, no tremor.

PSYCH: alert, oriented, cognitive function intact, cooperative with exam, good eye contact, judgment and insight good, speech clear, thought content without suicidal ideation, delusions.

ESR 30; CCP anti NL; HgBA1C 6.5; RA Factor 13.2; CBC WNL; lipid high, CMP WNL, ANA neg.

Critical Thinking:

1) What are the major concerns in this case?
2) What is your plan for Karla?
3) What teaching is appropriate at this time?

Mateo

HPI: Mateo is a 67-year-old Latino male who reports that he has tremors in his hands that have gotten worse. He works in a restaurant carrying heavy trays. His boss told him he's dropping too many things. Tremors are worse when he is working and decrease at rest; however, he has tremors with activity and at rest. He denies any slowing or stiffening of movements generally. He admits to increased fatigue. Mateo denies dizziness or difficulty with balance or coordination. He denies other tremors. He is not sleeping well. He reports he is taking his antihypertensives. He uses meloxicam with moderate relief of left shoulder pain.

Medications:

Meloxicam 7.5 mg 1 tablet orally twice a day.
Voltaren 1% gel as directed transdermal four times a day.
Hydrochlorothiazide 25 mg 1 tablet daily.
Vitamin D3 2000 unit capsule daily.

Medical/Surgical History:

Hyperlipidemia.
OA left shoulder.

FMH:

Father: deceased, colon cancer.
Mother: deceased, unknown cause.
Siblings are alive and well.
No children.

SH:

Denies use of alcohol, recreational drugs, or tobacco. Living with wife. Works full time as a waiter and bus boy.

Allergies: NKDA.

Vital Signs:

Ht 66 in, Wt 142 lbs, BP 124/72 mmHg, HR 84/min, RR 16/min, Temp 98.4 F.

General Examination:

GENERAL APPEARANCE: thin, frail, alert and oriented ×3, in no acute distress.
HEAD: normocephalic, atraumatic, no tremors of head or neck.
EYES: pupils equal, round, reactive to light and accommodation.
NECK/THYROID: neck supple, no cervical lymphadenopathy, no thyromegaly, thyroid nontender.
SKIN: warm and dry.
HEART: S1, S2 normal, regular rate and rhythm, no murmurs, rubs, gallops, no clicks.
LUNGS: clear to auscultation bilaterally.
EXTREMITIES: good capillary refill in nail beds, no clubbing, cyanosis, or edema.
PERIPHERAL PULSES: 2+ dorsalis pedis, 2+ posterior tibial, 2+ radial.
NEUROLOGIC: able to walk quickly and steadily down the hall. No apparent rigidity of movements, no slowing of movements. Slight tremor noted with hands at rest and with intention. No discoloration of hands or wrists, cerebellar function is normal, alert and oriented, cognitive exam is grossly normal, cooperative with exam, cranial nerves II–XII are grossly intact, deep tendon reflexes 2+ symmetrical, motor strength normal upper and lower extremities, no rigidity, strength 3/5 in BL hands.

PSYCH: alert, oriented, cognitive function intact, cooperative with exam, good eye contact, judgment and insight good, speech clear, thought content without suicidal ideation, delusions.

Critical Thinking:

1) What are the major concerns in this case?
2) What is your plan for Mateo?
3) What teaching is appropriate at this time?

Natalia

HPI: Natalia is a 40-year-old Russian female concerned about a possible infection in her bilateral thumbnails for six months. She recently developed pain and swelling, with erythema in the nail of the third digit of her left hand. She washes dishes at a restaurant all day but wears short gloves, so the water gets inside.

Medications:

Metformin HCL 500 mg 1 tablet with a meal once a day.
Lexapro 20 mg 1 tablet in the morning once a day.
Simvastatin 10 mg tablet, 1 tablet once a day.

Medical/Surgical History:

Prediabetes.
Depression with anxiety.

FMH:

Mother: deceased of unknown causes.
Father: alive, DMT2.
Five children: alive and well.
No siblings.

SH:

Denies use of tobacco, alcohol, or recreational drugs.

OB/GYN History:

Five pregnancies; five NSVD.
Periods: every month without discomfort/pain, light, lasts two to seve days.
Currently sexually active.
Last Pap smear: three years ago, negative.
Last mammogram: three years ago, bi-rad 1.
Sexually transmitted diseases: none.
Birth control: condoms.

Allergies: NKDA.

ROS:

HEENT: denies headaches.
Cardiovascular/respiratory: denies chest pain, dizziness, palpitations, pain with inspiration, shortness of breath at rest or with exertion.
GI/GU: denies abdominal pain, blood in stool or urine, change in bowel habits, difficulty urinating.
Psychiatric: anxiety and depression are controlled with Lexapro.

Vital Signs:

Ht 63 in, Wt 157 lbs, BP 118/76 mmHg, HR 64/min, RR 14/min, Temp 98.6 F.

General Examination:

GENERAL APPEARANCE: alert, well hydrated, in no distress.
EYES: pupils equal, round, reactive to light and accommodation, extraocular movement intact.
ORAL CAVITY: mucosa moist.
NECK/THYROID: no cervical lymphadenopathy, no thyroid nodules, no thyromegaly.
SKIN: BL thumbnails are hard, brittle, and discolored. Nail of third digit left hand is brittle, grooved. DIP is erythematous and swollen, no TTP.

HEART: S1, S2 normal, regular rate and rhythm, no murmurs, rubs, gallops, no clicks.

LUNGS: clear to auscultation bilaterally.

ABDOMEN: bowel sounds present, soft, nontender, nondistended, no hepatosplenomegaly, no guarding or rigidity.

EXTREMITIES: good capillary refill in nail beds, no clubbing, cyanosis, or edema.

PERIPHERAL PULSES: 2+ dorsalis pedis, 2+ posterior tibial, 2+ radial.

NEUROLOGIC: nonfocal, alert and oriented.

PSYCH: alert, oriented, cognitive function intact, cooperative with exam, good eye contact, judgment and insight good, speech clear, thought content without suicidal ideation, delusions.

Critical Thinking:

1) What are the major concerns in this case?
2) What is your plan for Natalia?
3) What should be included in patient teaching for Natalia?

Pedro

HPI: Pedro, a 67-year-old male Latino patient, presents for hand and knee pain.

Medications:

None.

Medical/Surgical History:

Denies chronic illness, hospitalizations, surgeries.

FMH:

Father: alive and well.
Mother: deceased age 60, DM.
Eleven siblings: alive and well.
Wife and two daughters are alive and well.

SH:

Denies use of tobacco, alcohol, recreational drugs.
Living with a friend. Married, but wife and children live in patient's home country. Occupation: works part time in a restaurant.

Allergies: NKDA.

ROS:

HEENT: denies headaches, problems with vision, dental problems.
Cardiovascular/respiratory: reports fluid accumulation in the legs after prolonged standing at work. Denies chest pain, dizziness, palpitations, hemoptysis, shortness of breath at rest or with exertion.
GI/GU: denies abdominal pain, blood in stool or urine, change in bowel habits. Reports nocturia ×4. Denies urinary incontinence.
Musculoskeletal: reports pain and swelling in both hands. He says he has had this problem for a long time; he sometimes drops things at work because his hands hurt. He also reports new bilateral knee pain. Pedro works at a restaurant carrying heavy trays. Pain is 7/10 and intermittent. He takes naproxen 200 mg and uses Voltaren gel with relief.
Neurologic: denies balance difficulty, gait abnormality.

Vital Signs:

Ht 64 in, Wt 154 lbs, BP 127/80 mmHg, HR 66/min, RR 14/min, Temp 97.8 F.

General Examination:

GENERAL APPEARANCE: alert, well hydrated, in no distress, pleasant, well nourished.
HEAD: normocephalic, atraumatic.
EYES: pupils equal, round, reactive to light and accommodation, extraocular movement intact, fundus normal, pink conjunctiva.
NECK/THYROID: no carotid bruit, carotid pulse normal, neck supple, full range of motion, no cervical lymphadenopathy, no jugular venous distention, no thyromegaly.
SKIN: good turgor, warm and dry, normal hair distribution.
HEART: S1, S2 normal, regular rate and rhythm, no murmurs, rubs, gallops, no clicks.

LUNGS: clear to auscultation bilaterally.

MUSCULOSKELETAL: FROM BL knees; Left hand: nodules across MCPs and thumb. Right hand: early nodule second digit MCP. No synovitis or erythema.

RECTAL: prostate is smooth and mildly enlarged. Guaiac is negative.

EXTREMITIES: no edema, good capillary refill in nail beds.

PERIPHERAL PULSES: 2+ dorsalis pedis, 2+ posterior tibial.

NEUROLOGIC: alert and oriented, cognitive exam grossly normal, cooperative with exam, deep tendon reflexes 2+ symmetrical, gait normal.

PSYCH: alert, oriented, cognitive function intact, cooperative with exam, good eye contact, speech clear.

Critical Thinking:

1) What are the major concerns in this case?
2) What is your plan for Pedro?
3) What teaching is appropriate at this time?

Regina

HPI: Regina, 50 years old, is a Latina female who presents following a telehealth visit with an endocrinologist during which she reported chest pain, radiation to her left arm, nausea, and diaphoresis. She denies vomiting. The pain first started eight days ago while working at Burger King. The episode lasted 20 minutes. Regina points to the LSB as the site of the pain. She says she became pale, so she sat down; colleagues gave her orange juice and sent her home. That evening, she ate garlic and the pain decreased. She eats garlic when she has chest pain, and that usually resolves the pain. She states that the current chest pain moves around from the LSB to different points in the left chest. She denies feeling nausea or having diaphoresis with the recent episodes. The current pain is intermittent, lasts approximately two hours each time, and typically occurs in the afternoon. Her typical diet includes water, orange juice, pancakes, and papusas. She makes her own food and denies eating at restaurants or elsewhere. She admits to feeling anxious at night.

Medications:

Not taking: methimazole 5 mg, 6 tablets once a day. Hydrochlorothiazide 25 mg 1 tablet in the morning once a day.

Medical/Surgical History:

Hyperthyroidism.
C-section 15 years ago.

FMH:

Father: deceased, homicide.
Mother: alive, high blood pressure.
Two sisters: alive and well. Three sons: alive and well.

SH:

Denies use of tobacco, alcohol, or recreational drugs.
Living with friends. Marital status: single. Occupation: full-time cashier at Burger King.

OB/GYN History:

Total pregnancies: three NSVD.
Periods: they were every month, but periods are starting to become further apart, approximately every two months. They last three to four days and are not heavy. Denies cramping.
Last Pap smear: three years ago. ASCUS with negative HPV low-volume reflex.
Last mammogram: one year ago, bi-rad 1.
Sexually transmitted diseases: none.
Birth control: bilateral tubal ligation.

Allergies: NKDA.

Vital Signs:

Ht 62 in, Wt 201 lbs, BP 158/89 mmHg, HR 88/min, RR 16min, Temp 98.1 F.

General Examination:

GENERAL APPEARANCE: alert, well hydrated, in no distress, well developed, well nourished, obese.

HEART: S1, S2 normal, regular rate and rhythm, no murmurs, rubs, gallops, no clicks. EKG: NSR.

LUNGS: clear to auscultation bilaterally.

ABDOMEN: BS are audible, no bruits, soft, NT, nondistended, no HSM, negative Murphy's sign. No guarding or rigidity.

EXTREMITIES: 1+ pitting edema lower extremities.

PERIPHERAL PULSES: 2+ dorsalis pedis, 2+ posterior tibial.

Regina is asked to restart methimazole per endocrinologist and to restart hydrochlorothiazide. She is asked to start omeprazole delayed release, 10 mg, 1 capsule 30 minutes before meals, twice a day, and to stop eating garlic and avoid spicy food. She should sit up for at least half an hour after eating. Weight loss will also help to reduce acid reflux.

She is given a BP cuff to record BP 3× / week (at rest) for the next two weeks and is asked to bring the record back to the next visit.

Regina RTC for follow-up in two weeks:

TSH, T3, and T4 are abnormal.

HPI: Regina presents for FU. Her BPs at home average 138–148/80s–90s. She states she does not sleep well because she is anxious. She has tried melatonin, but it makes her itch. Now, she is taking two Benadryl tablets at night. She denies epigastric or abdominal pain. She is not taking omeprazole. She reports pain in the lateral aspect of her left foot. She denies trauma; however, she stands a lot at work.

Medications:

Methimazole 5 mg tablet, 6 tablets once a day.
Hydrochlorothiazide 25 mg tablet, 1 tablet in the morning once a day.

ROS:

HEENT: denies headaches, problems with vision.

Cardiovascular/respiratory: denies chest pain, palpitations, dizziness, fluid accumulation in the legs, hemoptysis, pain with inspiration, shortness of breath at rest or with exertion.

Musculoskeletal: reports pain on lateral side of left foot.

Vital Signs:

BP 134/84 mmHg, HR 80/min, RR 16/min, Temp 98.7 F.

General Examination:

GENERAL APPEARANCE: in no acute distress, well developed, well nourished, cooperative.

HEART: regular rate and rhythm, no rubs, no murmurs, no clicks.

LUNGS: clear to auscultation bilaterally.

MUSCULOSKELETAL: moderate tenderness to palpation of the left foot on/near head of fifth metatarsal along lateral edge of midfoot. No bruising, edema, or discoloration. Full range of motion in bilateral ankles. Pain to resisted dorsiflexion of left foot.

EXTREMITIES: no gross deformity. Reflexes 2+. Palpable pedal pulses. Strength 5/5.

PERIPHERAL PULSES: +2 radial.

NEUROLOGIC: alert and oriented, cerebellar function normal, cognitive exam grossly normal, cooperative with exam, motor strength normal upper and lower extremities.

Test results:

Pap smear and pelvic exam reveal uterine prolapse.

X-ray foot left: negative.

Pelvic US: shows uterine prolapse.

Losartan potassium is added to the medication regimen. Regina is given a short course of trazodone to help her sleep. She should take half of a 50 mg tablet at bedtime.

Regina RTC in two weeks for follow-up:

HPI: Regina presents for FU. She is checking her BP at home and averaging 120s–130s/88–85. She is taking all of her medications (except for omeprazole), including trazodone for sleep. "I cannot sleep without it." She gets home from work at 11:30 p.m. two nights each week; on the other nights, she works all night and sleeps in the daytime. She says she must eat when she gets home at night or early in the morning before she sleeps because she doesn't have time to eat at work. She has had her period for two weeks with heavy bleeding and clots. She reports continued left foot pain. She stands on her feet for prolonged periods at work.

Medications:

Losartan potassium 25 mg 1 tablet orally once a day.
Methimazole 5 mg 8 tablets orally once a day.
Trazodone HCl 50 mg ½ tablet at bedtime as needed orally once a day.
Hydrochlorothiazide 25 mg 1 tablet in the morning orally once a day.
She is not taking omeprazole.

Vital Signs:

Ht 62 in, Wt 200 lbs, BP 128/76 mmHg, HR 80/min, RR 16/min, Temp 97.9 F.
GENERAL APPEARANCE: in no acute distress, well developed, well nourished, cooperative.
HEART: regular rate and rhythm, no rubs, no murmurs, no clicks.
LUNGS: clear to auscultation bilaterally.

Critical Thinking:

1) What are the major concerns in this case?
2) What is your plan for Regina?
3) What teaching is appropriate at this time?

6

Trauma/Mental Health Issues

Alba

HPI: Alba, age 29, presents for FU and review of blood work results. She reports stress related to being alone in this country from Latin America, losing her mother two years ago, breaking up with an abusive boyfriend after a four-year relationship three years ago after he went to jail, loans, and financial distress. Alba reports daily hair loss and forgetfulness. She is working with a lawyer to get a visa, but her lawyer anticipates this will take another two years to complete. Alba was advised not to go home until she has a visa or she will not be able to return to the United States. She was alone in her house all last year due to COVID-19 and was very depressed. She says she saw a psychiatrist weekly through telehealth and took medicine for two years but decided to stop it because it made her sleepy. She gets some comfort from church services and the people there, but she remains depressed. She denies SI or a wish to harm herself or others.

Medications:

None.

Medical/Surgical History:

None.

Caring for the Displaced and Uninsured: Clinical Case Studies in Nursing & Healthcare, First Edition. Leslie Neal-Boylan.
© 2023 John Wiley & Sons Ltd. Published 2023 by John Wiley & Sons Ltd.

FMH:

Mother: alive and well in home country.
Father: deceased age 60 from "kidney problems."
No partner or children.

Allergies: NKDA.

Vital Signs:

Ht 60 in, Wt 200 lbs, BP 118/76 mmHg, HR 84/min, RR 16/min, Temp 97.6 F.

General Examination:

GENERAL APPEARANCE: obese, alert, well hydrated, in no distress.
EYES: pupils equal, round, reactive to light and accommodation.
SKIN: warm and dry, lesions from removal of skin tags have healed. Mild
    erythema remains. No signs of infection, normal hair distribution, +
    acanthosis migrans.
HEART: S1, S2 normal, regular rate and rhythm, no murmurs, rubs, gal-
    lops, no clicks.
LUNGS: clear to auscultation bilaterally.
EXTREMITIES: good capillary refill in nail beds, no clubbing, cyanosis,
    or edema.
PERIPHERAL PULSES: 2+ radial.
NEUROLOGIC: nonfocal, alert and oriented.
PSYCH: alert, oriented, cognitive function intact, cooperative with exam,
    good eye contact, judgment and insight good, speech clear, thought
    content without suicidal ideation, delusions.
HgBA1C = 6.2 (5.8 two years ago).

Critical Thinking:

1) What are the major concerns in this case?
2) What is your plan for Alba?
3) What patient teaching is appropriate at this time?

Elena

HPI: Elena, 48-year-old Latina female, presents for FU of DMT2. She
states she feels well but needs medication refills.

Medications:

Losartan potassium 50 mg at oral daily.
Atorvastatin 40 mg daily.
Lexapro 20 mg daily.
Metformin HCL 1000 mg 1 tablet with a meal orally twice daily.
Novolin R 100 unit/ml, inject 8 units prebreakfast and 8 units predinner
subcutaneous daily.
Novolin N 100 unit/ml, inject 30 units in a.m. and 20 units in p.m. subcutaneous twice a day.

Medical/Surgical History:

Depression with anxiety.
DM.
Total hysterectomy.

FMH:

Father: deceased, murdered.
Mother: alive and well.
Husband is dead.
Two sons: alive and well.

SH:

Denies use of tobacco, alcohol, or recreational drugs.
Living with family. Widowed. Unemployed.
Elena reports that in her home country her husband was murdered, and
she was physically tortured.

OB/GYN History:

Pregnancies: two NSVD, live children.
Not currently sexually active.
Last Pap smear: two years ago, negative.
Last mammogram: two years ago, negative.
Postmenopausal due to total hysterectomy.
Sexually transmitted diseases: none.

Allergies: NKDA.

ROS:

HEENT: denies headaches, problems with vision, dental problems.

Cardiovascular/respiratory: denies chest pain, dizziness, fluid accumulation in the legs, palpitations, cough, hemoptysis, pain with inspiration, shortness of breath at rest or with exertion.

GI/GU: denies abdominal pain, blood in stool or urine, change in bowel habits, constipation, difficulty urinating.

Musculoskeletal: denies MSK pain.

Skin: denies skin problems/concerns.

Neurologic: denies tingling/numbness.

Psychiatric: denies anxiety, depressed mood; both are controlled with medication. Denies difficulty sleeping or loss of appetite.

Vital Signs:

Ht 63 in, Wt 172 lbs, BP 105/68 mmHg, HR 94/min, RR 16/min, Temp 97.6 F.

General Examination:

GENERAL APPEARANCE: alert, well hydrated, in no distress.

EYES: pupils equal, round, reactive to light and accommodation, extraocular movement intact.

ORAL CAVITY: mucosa moist.

NECK/THYROID: no cervical lymphadenopathy, no thyromegaly, no thyroid nodules, no jugular venous distention, neck supple, full range of motion.

SKIN: warm and dry.

HEART: S1, S2 normal, regular rate and rhythm, no murmurs, rubs, gallops, no clicks.

LUNGS: clear to auscultation bilaterally.

ABDOMEN: bowel sounds present, soft, nontender, nondistended, no hepatosplenomegaly, no guarding or rigidity.

EXTREMITIES: good capillary refill in nail beds, no clubbing, cyanosis, or edema.

PERIPHERAL PULSES: 2+ dorsalis pedis, 2+ posterior tibial, 2+ radial.

NEUROLOGIC: nonfocal, alert and oriented.

PODIATRIC: sensation to light touch grossly intact. No apparent calluses or lesions.

PSYCH: alert, oriented, cognitive function intact, cooperative with exam, good eye contact, speech clear, thought content without suicidal ideation, delusions.

Critical Thinking:

1) What are the major concerns in this case?
2) What is your plan for Elena?
3) What teaching is appropriate at this time?

Miguel

HPI: Miguel, a 60-year-old Latino male, is a new patient who presents with a few concerns. He would like to have his vision checked. He uses reading glasses. He also reports BL LBP. He says it feels like he gets swelling in his lower back. He cannot lift anything heavy without pain. Miguel fell in 1987 on his back on a concrete step. He had no pain until recently. Miguel is a painter and carpenter.

Medications:

None.

Medical/Surgical History:

Active TB (treated).

FMH:

Father: deceased, murdered.
Mother: alive, knee replacement.
Two brothers: murdered.
Unmarried, no children.

SH:

Denies use of tobacco, alcohol, or recreational drugs.
Miguel grew up in a Latin American country. Every morning from the age of 9, he was awakened at 5 a.m. to go to school until 1 p.m., then to work in a clothing factory until 7 p.m. making ladies clothing. He walked home with his father in the dark. He reports that he slept with "one eye open." Both his brothers were killed in his country. He came to the

United States at age 18. He worries about his mother, who still lives in his home country, because the area in which she lives still is dangerous.

ROS:

General: Miguel says he gets shaky if he doesn't eat.

HEENT: denies headaches. Reports vision is changing. Wears partial dentures and has some missing teeth. Reports dental pain.

Cardiovascular/respiratory: denies chest pain, dizziness, edema, palpitations, cough, hemoptysis, pain with inspiration, shortness of breath at rest or exertion.

GI/GU: denies abdominal pain, blood in stool or urine, change in bowel or bladder habits, constipation, sexual dysfunction.

Musculoskeletal: reports chronic low back pain.

Skin: reports dry skin that cracks. Uses sandpaper to scrape off calluses.

Neurologic: denies memory loss, tingling/numbness, tremors.

Psychiatric: denies anxiety, depressed mood, difficulty sleeping, loss of appetite.

Vital Signs:

Ht 67 in, Wt 163 lbs, BP 155/85 mmHg, HR 65/min, RR 16/min, Temp 97.5 F.

General Examination:

GENERAL APPEARANCE: thin, alert, well hydrated, in no distress.

HEAD: normocephalic, atraumatic.

EYES: pupils equal, round, reactive to light and accommodation, extraocular movement intact.

ORAL CAVITY: mucosa moist.

THROAT: no erythema, no exudate, pharynx normal.

NECK/THYROID: carotid pulse normal, no carotid bruit, neck supple, full range of motion, no cervical lymphadenopathy, no jugular venous distention, no thyroid nodules, no thyromegaly, thyroid nontender.

SKIN: warm and dry, good turgor.

HEART: S1, S2 normal, regular rate and rhythm, no murmurs, rubs, gallops, no clicks.

LUNGS: clear to auscultation bilaterally.

ABDOMEN: bowel sounds present, soft, nontender, nondistended, no hepatosplenomegaly, no guarding or rigidity.

BACK: no costovertebral angle tenderness, full range of motion, normal exam of spine, spine nontender to palpation.

MUSCULOSKELETAL: mild left and right LBP on elevation of left and right legs (one at a time). Negative SLR.

EXTREMITIES: good capillary refill in nail beds, no clubbing, cyanosis, or edema.

PERIPHERAL PULSES: 2+ dorsalis pedis, 2+ posterior tibial, 2+ radial.

NEUROLOGIC: nonfocal, alert and oriented, cerebellar function normal, cognitive exam grossly normal, cooperative with exam, cranial nerves II–XII grossly intact, gait normal, motor strength normal upper and lower extremities, neck supple, no rigidity, no tremor.

PSYCH: alert, oriented, cognitive function intact, cooperative with exam, good eye contact, judgment and insight good, speech clear, thought content without suicidal ideation, delusions.

Critical Thinking:

1) What are the major concerns in this case?
2) What is your plan for Miguel?
3) What teaching is appropriate at this time?

Darva

HPI: Darva, a 22-year-old Eastern European female, presents to the clinic as a new patient. She arrived in the United States from a small, remote village four months ago. She reports insomnia due to nightmares during which she sees graveyards and lit candles. She reports her mother died when she was very young. She was raised to believe that witchcraft killed her mother. Darva describes an incident about a month ago. She was talking to other people when, suddenly, she began to feel chills up her spine that moved up her neck and to the back of her head. She lost consciousness and was told that she was unconscious for an hour. When she awoke, she did not recognize anyone and felt like the room was spinning. These effects lasted about 20 minutes. She is afraid to sleep so she naps during the day and does not work. Darva believes she is going to die and that a witch possesses her body. She admits to feeling anxious and depressed. She arrived in the United States with a male partner who was verbally abusive. They broke up. She is now living with a girlfriend with whom she feels safe.

Medications:

None.

Medical/Surgical History:

None.

FMH:

Father, two sisters, and a brother are alive and well in her home country.
Mother: died, age 40, of unknown causes.
Grandparents: died of unknown causes.
No spouse or children.

SH:

Denies use of tobacco, alcohol, or recreational drugs.

OB/GYN History:

No pregnancies.
Not currently sexually active.
Last Pap smear: never.
Last mammogram: never.
Last normal period: three weeks ago. Periods are monthly, regular, last four to five days with the first two days consisting of heavy bleeding and cramping.
Sexually transmitted diseases: none.
Birth control: none.

Allergies: NKDA.

ROS:

General: Reports insomnia. Able to fall asleep but is awakened every night by nightmares. Takes one or two ½-hour naps during the day. Always fatigued. Reports decreased appetite without weight loss. Denies night sweats or heat or cold intolerance.

HEENT: denies headaches or vision changes. Denies dental pain or problems with her teeth. Never had vision or dental screenings.

Cardiovascular/respiratory: reports occasional palpitations associated with anxiety and feeling "scared all the time." Denies chest pain, dizziness, edema, cough, hemoptysis, pain with inspiration, shortness of breath at rest or exertion.

GI/GU: denies abdominal pain, blood in stool or urine, change in bowel or bladder habits, constipation, sexual dysfunction.

Musculoskeletal: denies pain or limited range of motion.

Skin: reports some hair loss. Denies changes to skin or nails.

Neurologic: denies memory loss, tingling/numbness, tremors.

Psychiatric: reports anxiety, depressed mood, difficulty sleeping, loss of appetite.

Vital Signs:

Ht 63 in, Wt 110 lbs, BP 120/70 mmHg, HR 66/min, RR 14/min, Temp 97.5 F.

General Examination:

GENERAL APPEARANCE: alert, well hydrated, anxious appearing.

HEAD: normocephalic, atraumatic.

EYES: pupils equal, round, reactive to light and accommodation, extraocular movement intact.

ORAL CAVITY: mucosa moist, dentition is good.

THROAT: no erythema, no exudate, pharynx normal.

NECK/THYROID: no cervical lymphadenopathy, no thyroid nodules, no thyromegaly, thyroid nontender.

SKIN: warm and dry, good turgor.

HEART: S1, S2 normal, regular rate and rhythm, no murmurs, rubs, gallops, no clicks.

LUNGS: clear to auscultation bilaterally.

ABDOMEN: bowel sounds present, soft, nontender, nondistended, no hepatosplenomegaly, no guarding or rigidity.

BACK: no costovertebral angle tenderness, full range of motion, normal exam of spine, spine nontender to palpation.

MUSCULOSKELETAL: FROM without pain.

EXTREMITIES: good capillary refill in nail beds, no clubbing, cyanosis, or edema.

PERIPHERAL PULSES: 2+ dorsalis pedis, 2+ posterior tibial, 2+ radial.

NEUROLOGIC: nonfocal, alert and oriented, cerebellar function normal, cognitive exam grossly normal, cooperative with exam, cranial nerves II–XII grossly intact, gait normal, motor strength normal upper and lower extremities, neck supple, no rigidity, no tremor.

PSYCH: alert, oriented, cognitive function intact, appears anxious, cooperative with exam, poor eye contact, speech clear, thought content without suicidal ideation.

Critical Thinking:

1) What are the major concerns in this case?
2) What is your plan for Darva?
3) What teaching is appropriate at this time?

7

Specialty Access Issues

Carlos

HPI: Carlos is a 70-year-old male visiting family from his home country in Latin America. He is a new patient reporting burning and pain in his right hip radiating down the leg for five months. He has had a burning sensation for one month. The pain wakes him at night. He was examined in his home country before emigrating to the United States. Carlos describes what sounds like a Doppler study; he was told it was negative and that he has "circulation problems." Carlos reports having had erythema of both lower legs and numbness in the plantar surfaces of both feet. He denies trauma, swelling, or edema. His pain is getting worse. Ibuprofen doesn't provide relief. He takes several showers daily because the cold water helps.

Medication:

Ibuprofen 400 mg every six hours.

Allergies: NKDA.

Medical/Surgical History:

Renal calculus, prostate resection.

Caring for the Displaced and Uninsured: Clinical Case Studies in Nursing & Healthcare, First Edition. Leslie Neal-Boylan.
© 2023 John Wiley & Sons Ltd. Published 2023 by John Wiley & Sons Ltd.

FMH:

Both parents are deceased from an MVA.
His nine children are alive and well.

SH:

Current nonsmoker, smoked for 20 years. Cannot quantify. Quit three years ago. Denies alcohol or recreational drug use. Married, unemployed.

ROS:

Cardiovascular/respiratory: denies chest pain, dizziness, hemoptysis, pain with inspiration, shortness of breath.

Vital Signs:

Ht 62 in, Wt 140 lbs, BP 134/62 mmHg, HR 60/min, RR 16/min, Temp 97.8 F.

General Examination:

GENERAL APPEARANCE: alert, well hydrated, in no distress, son accompanies Pt to help with translation.
EYES: pupils equal, round, reactive to light and accommodation, extraocular movement intact.
ORAL CAVITY: mucosa moist.
NECK/THYROID: mass on right neck, slightly movable, soft, regular borders, ~4 cm. Carotid pulse normal, no carotid bruit, no jugular venous distention, no thyroid nodules, no thyromegaly.
SKIN: warm and dry, brown (hemosiderin) patches along both LEs, good turgor.
CHEST: large, approximately 5 cm mass, round, immoveable on chest, more hard than soft, anterior to left breast and lateral to acromion process. No axillary LAD. There is slight erythema around the left areola, no masses or discoloration of either breast, no nipple discharge, no dimpling.
HEART: S1, S2 normal, regular rate and rhythm, no murmurs, rubs, gallops, no clicks.

LUNGS: clear to auscultation bilaterally.

ABDOMEN: bowel sounds present, soft, nontender, nondistended, no hepatosplenomegaly, no guarding or rigidity.

BACK: spine nontender to palpation, normal exam of spine.

MUSCULOSKELETAL: +SLR BL (but difficult to confirm because of language barrier even with translator). Patient has BL low back pain with elevation/extension of LEs and with flexion of knees BL. Pt reports pain in right knee on extension and flexion.

EXTREMITIES: no clubbing, cyanosis, or edema, good capillary refill in nail beds.

PERIPHERAL PULSES: 2+ dorsalis pedis, 2+ posterior tibial, 2+ radial.

NEUROLOGIC: nonfocal, alert and oriented, cooperative with exam, cognitive exam grossly normal, cranial nerves II–XII grossly intact, deep tendon reflexes 2+ symmetrical, motor strength normal upper and lower extremities, no rigidity, no tremor.

PODIATRIC: onychomycosis of all toenails, but feet are warm and without lesions, calluses, erythema.

PSYCH: alert, oriented, cognitive function intact, cooperative with exam, good eye contact, judgment and insight good, speech clear, thought content without suicidal ideation, delusions.

Carlos RTC for FU appointment two weeks later:

HPI: Carlos says gabapentin has not helped numbness in BL LEs. He denies fever and chills. He feels generally well other than numbness in BL LEs. He is wearing compression stockings and walking daily.

Vital Signs:

BP 124/66 mmHg, HR 70/min, RR 16/min, Temp 98.4 F.

X-ray of L-S spine showed mild OA of BL hips, right SI, and symphysis pubis.

The clinician decides to increase gabapentin to 300 mg morning and afternoon and 400 mg at night. She refers the patient to a vascular surgeon. Carlos should stop the aspirin and take Tylenol for pain. Carlos is referred to vision screening.

CT chest, abdomen, and pelvis and ultrasound of neck reveal metastatic lung cancer.

The clinician calls the patient but is asked to speak with his son because the son speaks English.Carlos follows up two weeks later:

HPI: Carlos was informed by his son that he has lung cancer following the call from the clinician. They RTC today to learn more about the diagnosis and the results of the CT scan. Carlos continues to have pain in LLE and now has pain in the left abdomen. He tried Percocet once, felt dizzy and tired, so he stopped taking it. Carlos plans to stay in the United States.

Vital Signs:

Wt 138 lbs, BP 140/71 mmHg, HR 73/min, RR 16/min, Temp 98.2 F.

Lung and Liver Cancer:

The oncology office nearby has agreed to work with this patient although he is visiting this country and has no insurance. Their staff is reviewing the clinic records prior to scheduling an appointment. Via an interpreter, the PCP explains the diagnoses. They also discuss pain management. The patient or his son is to inform the PCP if the patient's appetite or sleep change. Carlos agrees to try ½ tablet of Percocet when he has pain so he can adjust to the side effects of sleepiness and mild dizziness. He will report unpleasant side effects. The PCP explains that the chronic right leg pain is most likely due to pressure from the mass on the liver.

Critical Thinking:

1) What are the major concerns in this case?
2) What is your plan for Carlos?
3) What teaching is appropriate at this time?

Sergio

HPI: Sergio, age 81, presents to establish primary care. He is accompanied by his adult son, who translates. He has been seeing an endocrinologist for DMT2 at the National Institutes of Health (NIH) as part of a clinical study. He was referred there last year by an urgent care provider. Sergio reports that his fasting blood sugars (FBG) have been in the 130s.

He denies signs and symptoms of hypoglycemia but reports the recent onset of dizziness, fatigue, and LE edema. He reports abdominal pain when he doesn't have a bowel movement for two days. He has been taking apple pectin, which relieves constipation and pain. He denies CP, dyspnea, or cough.

Medications:

Metformin 1000 mg 1 tablet twice a day, with meals.
Amlodipine besylate 10 mg 1 tablet once a day.
Hydrochlorothiazide 25 mg 1 tablet once a day.
Glipizide 10 mg 1 tablet in a.m. 30 minutes prebreakfast, 1 tablet in p.m. 30 minutes predinner.

Medical/Surgical History:

Diabetes mellitus type 2.
Hypertension.
Hyperlipidemia.

FMH:

Mother: deceased, alcoholism.
Father: deceased, stroke.
One son deceased from fall from roof while working. One son is alive and well.

SH:

Smoked as a teenager but none since. Drinks two 12-oz beers twice/week. Living with an adult son, widowed, unemployed.

ROS:

HEENT: denies headaches, problems with vision.
Cardiovascular/respiratory: admits to fluid accumulation in the legs. Denies chest pain, palpitations, pain with inspiration, shortness of breath at rest or with exertion.
Gastrointestinal: admits to intermittent constipation. LNBM this morning. Denies abdominal pain today, blood in stool, change in bowel habits, nausea or vomiting.

Genitourinary: denies abdominal pain/swelling, blood in urine, difficulty urinating.

Musculoskeletal: denies joint stiffness, painful joints.

Skin: denies dry skin, changing moles, rash.

Neurologic: admits to dizziness × two weeks—feeling like the room is spinning. Drinks four glasses of water daily. Denies memory changes, tingling/numbness.

Psychiatric: denies anxiety, depressed mood.

Vital Signs:

Ht 65 in, Wt 145 lbs, BP 170/86, HR 64/min, RR 16/min, Temp 98.2 F.

General Examination:

GENERAL APPEARANCE: alert, well hydrated, in no distress, does not usually make eye contact, defers to son.

EYES: pupils equal, round, reactive to light and accommodation, extraocular movement intact.

SKIN: warm and dry.

HEART: S1, S2 normal, regular rate and rhythm, no murmurs, rubs, gallops, no clicks.

LUNGS: clear to auscultation bilaterally.

EXTREMITIES: good capillary refill in nail beds, no clubbing, cyanosis, or edema.

PERIPHERAL PULSES: 2+ dorsalis pedis, 2+ posterior tibial, 2+ radial.

NEUROLOGIC: nonfocal, alert and oriented, cerebellar function intact, CNs II–XII grossly intact, DTRs +2.

Critical Thinking:

1) What are the major concerns in this case?
2) What is your plan for Sergio?
3) What teaching is appropriate at this time?

Valeria

HPI: Valeria, 38-year-old Eastern European female, presents with concerns about left breast pain and pelvic pain. She reports increasing left breast pain for three months. She reports pain when she elevates her left arm. She denies CP or dyspnea. She has a history of breast implants.

Her LMP, one month ago, was a bit heavier than usual for the first two days, with large clots. She does not think she can be pregnant. She does not like sexual intercourse because she has pelvic pain all the time, for which she is taking Tylenol with codeine she obtained from a friend. She denies bowel or bladder changes. Valeria expresses concern that she has cancer and fear that she will die and leave her children alone.

Medications:

Tylenol with codeine prn pain.

Medical/surgical history:

Breast implants.
Cholecystectomy.

FMH:

Her parents are alive and well in her home country in Eastern Europe.
Her two children are alive and well.

SH:

Nonsmoker. Drinks one 12-oz beer once a month. Denies recreational drug use.
Single. Employed part time as a housecleaner.

OB/GYN History:

One pregnancy. One NSVD.
Mammogram: none.
Pap smear: none.
Periods: every month regular. Does not remember date of last period.
Not currently sexually active.
Sexually transmitted diseases: none.
Birth control: none.

Allergies: NKDA.

Vital Signs:

Ht 64 in, Wt 165 lbs, BP 128/80 mmHg, HR 98/min, RR 16/min, Temp 96.8 F.

General Examination:

GENERAL APPEARANCE: alert and oriented ×3, very tearful.

HEAD: normocephalic, atraumatic.

EYES: pupils equal, round, reactive to light and accommodation.

HEART: S1, S2 normal, regular rate and rhythm, no murmurs, rubs, gallops, no clicks.

LUNGS: clear to auscultation bilaterally.

BREAST: axillary nodes normal; left breast: visible swelling in LUQ, no erythema, no dimpling, no swollen veins/varicosities, no nipple dc. LUQ mass is the size of a golf ball. Very tender to palpation. Right breast is soft, without masses, dimpling, or dc.

Critical Thinking:

1) What are the major concerns in this case?
2) What is your plan for Valeria?
3) What teaching is appropriate at this time?

8

Delayed Screening

Aurora

HPI: Aurora, age 52 years, is a new female patient who reports having a goiter. She says she had a goiter while in elementary school in the Philippines. She was given medicine ("two yellowish white pills, the size of my fingertip"), and the goiter went away. She has noticed the return of the goiter. Her last medical visit was five years ago in the United States for the birth of her last child.

Medications:

None.

Medical/Surgical History:

Goiter.
Appendectomy.

FMH:

Mother: deceased, stroke age 72.
Father: age 74, alive and well.

SH:

Denies use of tobacco, alcohol, or recreational drugs.
Living with boyfriend and three children, works full time as a housekeeper and nanny.

Caring for the Displaced and Uninsured: Clinical Case Studies in Nursing & Healthcare, First Edition. Leslie Neal-Boylan.
© 2023 John Wiley & Sons Ltd. Published 2023 by John Wiley & Sons Ltd.

OB/GYN History:

Three pregnancies. Three living children, NSVD.
Periods: irregular, every other month.
Currently sexually active.
Last Pap smear: six years ago, negative.
Never had a mammogram.

Allergies: NKDA.

ROS:

General/constitutional: denies change in appetite, sleep disturbance,
weight gain or loss.
HEENT: denies headaches or difficulty swallowing.
Endocrine: denies cold or heat intolerance.
Cardiovascular/respiratory: denies chest pain, dizziness, palpitations,
pain with inspiration, shortness of breath at rest or with exertion.
Psychiatric: denies anxiety or depression.

Vital Signs:

Ht 63 in, Wt 122 lbs, BP 146/87 mmHg, HR 66/min, RR 16/min, Temp 98.4 F.

General Examination:

GENERAL APPEARANCE: alert, well hydrated, in no distress.
EYES: pupils equal, round, reactive to light and accommodation, extraoc-
ular movement intact.
ORAL CAVITY: mucosa moist.
NECK/THYROID: moderate-sized swelling (size of golf ball), soft, in
right lobe of thyroid, NT. No bruit.
SKIN: warm and dry, normal hair distribution.
HEART: S1, S2 normal, regular rate and rhythm, no murmurs, rubs, gal-
lops, no clicks.
LUNGS: clear to auscultation bilaterally.
EXTREMITIES: good capillary refill in nail beds, no clubbing, cyanosis,
or edema.
PERIPHERAL PULSES: 2+ dorsalis pedis, 2+ posterior tibial,
2+ radial.

NEUROLOGIC: nonfocal, alert and oriented, deep tendon reflexes 2+ symmetrical, no rigidity, no tremor.

PSYCH: alert, oriented, cognitive function intact, cooperative with exam, good eye contact, judgment and insight good, speech clear, thought content without suicidal ideation, delusions.

Critical Thinking:

1) What are the major concerns in this case?
2) What is your plan for Aurora?
3) What teaching is appropriate at this time?

Mirikit

HPI: Mirikit, age 55, is a new patient who presents with high blood pressure for five years, since having a D&C in the Philippines. She has not had medical care since then. She takes valsartan and amlodipine that she gets from the Philippines. She takes vitamins B_{12} and D but has not been diagnosed with any deficiencies.

Medications:

Amlodipine 10 mg daily.
Valsartan 40 mg daily.

Medical/Surgical History:

FMH:

Parents are deceased, causes unknown.
Two daughters: alive and well.

SH:

Denies use of tobacco, alcohol, or recreational drugs.
Living with friends, married. Works full time as a housekeeper.

OB/GYN History:

Two pregnancies; two NSVD.
Not currently sexually active.

Last Pap smear: five years ago, abnormal.
Never had a mammogram.
Postmenopausal.
Sexually transmitted diseases: none.
Birth control: tubal ligation.
Fibroid uterus found on ultrasound.

Allergies: NKDA.

Vital Signs:

Ht 60 in, Wt 127 lbs, BP 172/98 mmHg, HR 118/min, RR 16/min, Temp 98.5 F.

General Examination:

GENERAL APPEARANCE: alert, well hydrated, in no distress.
HEAD: normocephalic, atraumatic.
EYES: pupils equal, round, reactive to light and accommodation, extraocular movement intact.
NECK/THYROID: no cervical lymphadenopathy, no jugular venous distention, no thyroid nodules, no thyromegaly.
SKIN: warm and dry.
HEART: grade I systolic murmur, regular rate and rhythm, no clicks.
LUNGS: clear to auscultation bilaterally.
EXTREMITIES: good capillary refill in nail beds, no clubbing, cyanosis, or edema.
PERIPHERAL PULSES: 2+ dorsalis pedis, 2+ posterior tibial, 2+ radial.
NEUROLOGIC: nonfocal, alert and oriented.
PSYCH: alert, oriented, cognitive function intact, cooperative with exam, good eye contact, judgment and insight good, speech clear, thought content without suicidal ideation, delusions.

Critical Thinking:

1) What are the major concerns in this case?
2) What is your plan for Mirikit?
3) What patient teaching is appropriate at this time?

9

Visitors

Franz

HPI: Franz is a 67-year-old self-pay male patient who presents as a new patient from Germany. He is living here with his wife, who works in the United States. He is unable to return home due to the COVID-19 pandemic. He has private insurance in Germany and needs medication refills. He reports his home BP as averaging 112/74.

Medications:

Sildenafil citrate 100 mg 1 tablet as needed daily.
Lisinopril 5 mg 1 tablet daily.

Medical/Surgical History:

HTN.
Erectile dysfunction.
Appendectomy.

FMH:

Both parents deceased of heart disease in their 70s.
One son: alive and well.
Wife: age 62, alive and well.

Caring for the Displaced and Uninsured: Clinical Case Studies in Nursing & Healthcare, First Edition. Leslie Neal-Boylan.
© 2023 John Wiley & Sons Ltd. Published 2023 by John Wiley & Sons Ltd.

SH:

Smoked for 20 years. Quit 10 years ago. Drinks two 16-oz beers on week-
end days. Denies use of recreational drugs.
Living with wife. Franz is a retired scientist.
Currently sexually active.
Sexually transmitted diseases: none.

ROS:

HEENT: denies headaches. Has prescription glasses for reading and dis-
tance. Denies dental problems. He sees a dentist regularly.
Cardiovascular/respiratory: denies chest pain, dizziness, palpitations.
Admits to fluid accumulation in the legs. Denies hemoptysis, pain
with inspiration, shortness of breath at rest or with exertion.
GI/GU: denies abdominal pain, blood in stool or urine, change in bowel
habits, constipation, difficulty urinating.
Musculoskeletal: denies joint stiffness, painful joints, swollen joints.
Skin: denies problems with hair, skin, nails. Had skin cancer lesion
removed from right temple, two years ago in Germany.
Neurologic: denies tingling/numbness, tremor.
Psychiatric: denies anxiety, depressed mood, difficulty sleeping, loss of
appetite.

Vital Signs:

Ht 72 in, Wt 220 lbs, BP 160/88 mmHg, HR 78/min, RR 16/min,
Temp 98.4 F.

General Examination:

GENERAL APPEARANCE: alert, well hydrated, in no distress.
HEAD: normocephalic, atraumatic.
EYES: pupils equal, round, reactive to light and accommodation, extraoc-
ular movement intact.
EARS: tympanic membrane intact, clear.
ORAL CAVITY: mucosa moist.
NECK/THYROID: carotid pulse normal, no carotid bruit, no cervical
lymphadenopathy, no jugular venous distention, no thyroid nodules,
no thyromegaly.

SKIN: scattered seborrheic keratosis throughout neck, chest, back, warm and dry.

HEART: S1, S2 normal, regular rate and rhythm, no murmurs, rubs, gallops, no clicks.

LUNGS: clear to auscultation bilaterally.

ABDOMEN: bowel sounds present, soft, nontender, nondistended, no hepatosplenomegaly, no guarding or rigidity.

BACK: full range of motion, no costovertebral angle tenderness, normal exam of spine, spine nontender to palpation.

MUSCULOSKELETAL: cervical spine normal, full range of motion, full range of motion of the hip, lumbosacral spine normal, no swelling or deformity.

EXTREMITIES: good capillary refill in nail beds, no clubbing, cyanosis, or edema, full range of motion.

PERIPHERAL PULSES: 2+ dorsalis pedis, 2+ posterior tibial, 2+ radial.

NEUROLOGIC: nonfocal, alert and oriented, cerebellar function normal, cognitive exam grossly normal, cooperative with exam, deep tendon reflexes 2+ symmetrical, motor strength normal upper and lower extremities, neck supple, no rigidity, no tremor.

PSYCH: alert, oriented, cognitive function intact, cooperative with exam, good eye contact, judgment and insight good, speech clear, thought content without suicidal ideation, delusions.

Critical Thinking:

1) What are the major concerns in this case?
2) What is your plan for Franz?
3) What patient teaching is appropriate at this time?

Marcos

HPI: Marcos is an 80-year-old male patient returning to the clinic after three years requesting medication refills. He takes Xarelto but doesn't know the dosage or the names of his other medications nor his health history. He lives in Latin America but is visiting here for six months and needs refills. He has not brought any of his medications or medical records. His son, who is present, says he cannot get records from the medical provider in his country.

Medications:

Unknown.

Medical/Surgical History:

Hypertension.

FMH:

Parents deceased. Mother had cancer of unknown type.
Father: cause of death or medical history unknown.
Siblings are alive and well.
No current spouse or partner. One son is alive and well.

SH:

Denies use of tobacco, alcohol, or recreational drugs.
Widowed and unemployed.

Vital Signs:

Ht 60 in, Wt 148 lbs, BP 150/85 mmHg, HR 118/min, RR 16/min,
Temp 98.6 F, Oxygen sat % 97%.

General Examination:

GENERAL APPEARANCE: alert, well hydrated, in no distress.
The visit is discontinued because the patient did not bring any medical
records and does not know his medical history.

The patient's son calls back later in the day and lists the patient's medications:

Valsartan 40 mg tablet, 1 tablet orally once a day.
Aspirin EC 81 mg tablet, delayed release 1 tablet orally once a day.
Lisinopril 20 mg tablet, 1 tablet orally once a day.
Amlodipine 5 mg 1 tablet orally daily.
Simvastatin 20 mg 1 tablet orally at night,
Hydrochlorothiazide 25 mg 1 tablet orally once a day.

Critical Thinking:

1) What are the major concerns in this case?
2) What is your plan for Marcos?
3) What teaching is appropriate at this time?

Trang

HPI: Trang, an 82-year-old Vietnamese man, presents with his son to translate. He has been visiting in the United States for one year and hopes to go home soon. Two weeks ago, his son took him to the ED because he had left-sided weakness, ptosis of the left eye, and the left side of his lower lip drooped. It had been four years since his last medical visit. He had never been diagnosed with HTN, hyperlipidemia, DM, or any other chronic disease. He had not been taking any medication prior to the ED visit. He drinks ginseng tea and takes one tablet of ginkgo biloba daily. In the hospital, Trang was diagnosed with a CVA and put on rosuvastatin and baby aspirin. The son cannot recall being given a prescription for an antihypertensive medication. He couldn't reach anyone when he called back to the hospital. The patient's son obtained lisinopril from a friend and initially gave Trang 50 mg. Two hours later, he gave the patient another 25 mg. The son wants to send Trang back to Vietnam to his home as soon as possible. The patient would like to go home.

Imaging and lab tests were performed in the hospital. The results are below:

CXR: enlarged heart size, atherosclerotic aorta, diffuse DJD of thoracic spine, DJD OA of BL shoulders.
MRA of brain: no large vessel occlusion. No aneurysm.
MRA of neck: no occlusion. No carotid or vertebral artery stenosis.
MRI brain: acute infarction in right caudate head—ischemic infarct.
CT head: microvascular changes.
CT brain perfusion: no acute ischemia or infarct.
CBC WNL.
Lipids: HDL 42/LDL 133.

Medications:

MVI daily.
Ginkgo biloba 120 mg tablet daily.
Lisinopril 75 mg 1 tablet once a day.
Rosuvastatin 20 mg 1 tablet once a day.
Aspirin 81 mg 1 tablet once a day.

Medical/Surgical History:

CVA—right infarction.
HTN.

FMH:

Father: deceased, sudden death at 59 years.
Mother: deceased, cause of death unknown, age 80.
One son, age 45, alive and well.

SH:

Smoked cigars but quit 10 years ago. Drinks 1–2 glasses of red or white
wine 4 times per week. Living with son. Retired.

ROS:

HEENT: denies headaches. Eyes: Trang reports difficulty with vision
before and since CVA.
Cardiovascular/respiratory: denies chest pain, dizziness, fluid accumulation in legs, palpitations. Denies cough, hemoptysis, pain with inspiration, shortness of breath at rest or with exertion.
GI/GU: denies abdominal pain, blood in stool or urine, change in bowel
habits, difficulty urinating.
Musculoskeletal: Pt denies joint stiffness, swollen joints, painful joints,
weakness. Trang can receive only one visit each from PT, OT, and ST
because he has no insurance. He is using a rolling walker.
Neurologic: denies memory loss, tingling/numbness, tremors.
The son started checking Trang's BP at home. BPs average 144/98 before
taking lisinopril and 110/60 one hour after taking lisinopril. Trang did
not take his medicine today.

Vital Signs:

Ht 67 in, Wt 145 lbs, BP 152/78 mmHg, HR 78/min, RR 16/min, Temp 98.7 F.

General Examination:

GENERAL APPEARANCE: frail-appearing male, alert and oriented, well hydrated, in no acute distress. Sitting with arms resting on walker.

HEAD: normocephalic, atraumatic.

EYES: BL arcus senilis, mild ptosis left upper eyelid, extraocular movement intact.

EARS: BL hearing aids.

ORAL CAVITY: mucosa moist.

THROAT: no erythema, no exudate, pharynx normal.

NECK/THYROID: no cervical lymphadenopathy, no jugular venous distention, no thyroid nodules, no thyromegaly.

SKIN: warm and dry, normal hair distribution.

HEART: S1, S2 normal, regular rate and rhythm, no murmurs, rubs, gallops, no clicks.

LUNGS: clear to auscultation bilaterally.

MUSCULOSKELETAL: no swelling or deformity, strength 5/5 and equal in both UEs and LEs. Strong BL hand grip. Walks steadily using rolling walker.

EXTREMITIES: good capillary refill in nail beds, no clubbing, cyanosis, or edema, walks steadily in hallway. No limping or favoring of left side.

PERIPHERAL PULSES: 2+ dorsalis pedis, 2+ posterior tibial, 2+ radial.

NEUROLOGIC: Trang says he is unsure why he went to the hospital, saying: "I feel normal." He is not sure why he is here today. He appears to think he is still in the hospital. Trang asked his son if this visit completes his hospital stay. The son says he recognizes people but doesn't remember their names. This was not a problem prior to the CVA. Trang can identify the year but is unable to identify the month or day.

PSYCH: cooperative with exam, good eye contact, speech clear.

The clinician explains to Trang's son that Trang's stroke could have caused impairment in judgment. Trang may not be safe alone. She asks the son not to give the patient medications without consulting her and to stop ginkgo biloba because it is a blood thinner. Ginseng may be raising his blood pressure. Trang should continue taking rosuvastatin in the evening and the baby aspirin daily. Trang is not ready to undertake a very long trip back to Vietnam. Trang is a self-pay patient, so the son is given a list of neurologists to call to try to schedule an appointment. Lisinopril is decreased to 20 mg/day.

Critical Thinking:

1) What are the major concerns in this case?
2) What is your plan for Trang?
3) What teaching is appropriate at this time?

10

Immigration Issues

Gabriela

HPI: Gabriela is a 38-year-old Latina female who presents as a new patient for a PE and treatment for hypothyroidism. Gabriela spent one year in an immigration detention center in Dallas, TX. She was told she had something wrong with her thyroid and was given medicine, sometimes 25 "milligrams," sometimes 50. She has not had any medicine for six months.

Medications:

None.

Medical/Surgical History:

Hypothyroidism.

FMH:

Father: alive, family history unknown.
Mother: alive, family history unknown.
Four children: alive and well.

SH:

Denies use of tobacco, alcohol, or recreational drugs. Living with sister, married, and husband lives in home country. She works part time in a cleaning job.

Caring for the Displaced and Uninsured: Clinical Case Studies in Nursing & Healthcare, First Edition. Leslie Neal-Boylan.
© 2023 John Wiley & Sons Ltd. Published 2023 by John Wiley & Sons Ltd.

OB/GYN History:

Four pregnancies. Four living children.
Periods: every month.
Currently sexually active.
Last Pap smear three years ago: negative.
Sexually transmitted diseases: none.
Birth control: none.

Allergies: NKDA.

ROS:

General/constitutional: denies chills, fever, fatigue.
HEENT: denies headaches. Reports occasional blurry vision. She reports broken teeth. She has pain with hot and cold foods.
Endocrine: reports hair loss. She denies heat or cold intolerance.
Cardiovascular: admits dizziness, drinks a lot of water, but eats once/day.
GI/GU: she has epigastric pain no matter what she eats and then becomes nauseous and vomits. She reports a burning sensation until she vomits. She has had these symptoms for one month and reports losing five pounds. Admits to nausea, vomiting, abdominal pain, and blood in the stool. Denies blood in urine or difficulty urinating, constipation, diarrhea, or heartburn.
Psychiatric: denies anxiety. Admits to loss of appetite and depressed mood, because her children are in her home country. She has two sisters here. Admits to difficulty sleeping; exercising helps.

Vital Signs:

Ht 62.5 in, Wt 104 lbs, BP 106/64 mmHg, HR 78/min, RR 14/min, Temp 98.6 F.

General Examination:

GENERAL APPEARANCE: slim, alert, well hydrated, in no distress.
HEAD: normocephalic, atraumatic.
EYES: pupils equal, round, reactive to light and accommodation, extraocular movement intact.
EARS: tympanic membrane intact, clear.

ORAL CAVITY: mucosa moist, poor dentition, all bottom teeth appear decayed.

THROAT: no erythema, no exudate.

NECK/THYROID: no cervical lymphadenopathy, no jugular venous distention, no thyroid nodules, no thyromegaly, thyroid nontender.

SKIN: warm and dry, normal hair distribution, no suspicious lesions.

HEART: S1, S2 normal, regular rate and rhythm, no murmurs, rubs, gallops, no clicks.

LUNGS: clear to auscultation bilaterally.

ABDOMEN: bowel sounds present, soft, nontender, nondistended, no hepatosplenomegaly, no guarding or rigidity.

BACK: full range of motion, no costovertebral angle tenderness, normal exam of spine, spine nontender to palpation.

MUSCULOSKELETAL: cervical spine normal, full range of motion, full range of motion of the hip, lumbosacral spine normal, no swelling or deformity.

EXTREMITIES: full range of motion, good capillary refill in nail beds, no clubbing, cyanosis, or edema.

PERIPHERAL PULSES: 2+ dorsalis pedis, 2+ posterior tibial, 2+ radial.

NEUROLOGIC: nonfocal, alert and oriented, cerebellar function normal, cognitive exam grossly normal, cooperative with exam, cranial nerves II–XII grossly intact, deep tendon reflexes 2+ symmetrical, gait normal, motor strength normal upper and lower extremities, neck supple, no rigidity, no tremor.

PSYCH: alert, oriented, cognitive function intact, cooperative with exam, good eye contact, judgment and insight good, speech clear, thought content without suicidal ideation, delusions.

Critical Thinking:

1) What are the major concerns in this case?
2) What is your plan for Gabriela?
3) What teaching is appropriate at this time?

Isabella

HPI: Isabella, a 25-year-old female, reports feeling anxious. She has been in the United States for one year, having left her home country due to violence and people trying to hurt her and her child. She states she thinks about it a lot. She denies any trigger regarding why she is anxious now. She says she has felt this way for a while. She reports palpitations and mild dizziness. She is taking medicine for anxiety from her home country. She cannot remember the name. She is currently lactating and not using any birth control.

Medication:

Unknown anxiety medicine.

Medical/Surgical History:

Anxiety.

FMH:

Parents and children are alive and well. Pt has no spouse or partner.

SH:

Denies use of tobacco, alcohol, or recreational drugs. Single, living with parents, unemployed.

OB/GYN History:

Two pregnancies. One NSVD and one Cesarean section; two living children, ages four years and four months.
Last Pap smear: one year ago, negative.
Date of last period: irregular, LNMP was two months ago.
Not currently sexually active.
Sexually transmitted diseases: none.
Birth control: none.

Allergies: NKDA.

ROS:

HEENT: reports myopia. Last saw an eye doctor in her home country two years ago. Does not wear glasses or contacts. Denies headaches, nasal congestion, sinus pain, dental problems, sore throat, or dysphagia. Last saw dentist two years ago in home country.

Cardiovascular/respiratory: denies chest pain, palpitations, dizziness, cough, hemoptysis, pain with inspiration, shortness of breath at rest or with exertion.

GI/GU: denies abdominal pain, blood in stool or urine, change in bowel habits, difficulty urinating, urgency, or frequency. Women only: reports BL pelvic pain. Reports missed periods last two months; had a period one month after delivery, none since. Denies painful intercourse.

Musculoskeletal: denies pain or limited mobility.

Skin: Pt denies concerns about skin, hair, or nails.

Psychiatric: reports intermittent anxiety, especially at night. Her thoughts keep her awake. When she finally falls asleep, the baby wakes her. Reports constant fatigue.

Vital Signs:

Ht 61 in, Wt 150 lb 6 oz, BP 120/80 mmHg, HR 70/min, RR 16/min, Temp 98.8 F.

General Examination:

GENERAL APPEARANCE: alert, well hydrated, in no distress, well nourished.

HEAD: normocephalic, atraumatic.

EYES: pupils equal, round, reactive to light and accommodation.

NECK/THYROID: neck supple, full range of motion, no cervical lymphadenopathy, no thyromegaly.

HEART: S1, S2 normal, regular rate and rhythm, no murmurs, rubs, gallops, no clicks.

LUNGS: clear to auscultation bilaterally.

ABDOMEN: bowel sounds present, soft, nontender, nondistended, no hepatosplenomegaly.

MUSCULOSKELETAL: full range of motion.

EXTREMITIES: good capillary refill in nail beds, no edema.

PERIPHERAL PULSES: 2+ dorsalis pedis, 2+ posterior tibial.

NEUROLOGIC: alert and oriented, cognitive exam grossly normal, cooperative with exam, cranial nerves II–XII grossly intact, deep tendon reflexes 2+ symmetrical, gait normal, motor strength normal upper and lower extremities.

PSYCH: alert, oriented, cognitive function intact, cooperative with exam, good eye contact, speech clear.

Critical Thinking:

1) What are the major concerns in this case?
2) What is your plan for Isabella?
3) What teaching is appropriate at this time?

Ivanna

HPI: Ivanna is a 20-year-old female who presents with severe pain in both wrists and at the base of each thumb R > L. She wears CTS splints at night and takes naproxen with a little relief. She denies trauma. Ivanna arrived in the United States last spring. She says she walked most of the way from Honduras, through Guatemala and Mexico. She came alone, occasionally walking with people she met along the way. Her family and friends remain in her home country. She has no one here. She is working part time cleaning businesses. She also reports LBP, especially on the right side for five months. She denies carrying heavy things.

Medication:

Naproxen 250 mg 1 tablet with food or milk as needed every 12 hours.

Medical/Surgical History:

CTS.

FMH:

Parents: medical history unknown. Both are alive.
One sister: alive and well.

SH:

Ivanna says she sometimes smokes, not every day. She cannot quantify how many cigarettes she smokes on an average day. She drinks beer two to four times per month, typically two 16-oz bottles. She admits to having used painkillers and sleep medications in the past year but doesn't know the names of the medications.
She is living alone in a shelter; she is single.

OB/GYN History:

No pregnancies.

Periods: irregular, she took Depo-Provera shots before her trip so she wouldn't get her period. Periods have not returned to regular monthly cycle although she stopped taking Depo-Provera two months ago.

LMP: four months ago

Allergies: NKDA.

ROS:

HEENT: reports occasional headaches, approximately once/month. Ivanna is nearsighted. She had glasses in her home country, but they broke, and she cannot afford to replace them. She denies dental problems but needs screening.

Cardiovascular/respiratory: admits to chest pain at rest, when she is sad or tired. Denies chest pain with exertion, dizziness, fluid accumulation in the legs, palpitations, cough, hemoptysis, pain with inspiration, shortness of breath at rest or with exertion.

GI/GU: denies abdominal pain, blood in stool or urine, change in bowel or bladder habits, constipation, heartburn, nausea, vomiting.

Skin: reports she has been losing hair. Denies problems with skin and nails.

Neurologic: admits to tingling/numbness in BL wrists.

Psychiatric: denies anxiety, depressed mood. Admits to difficulty sleeping.

Vital Signs:

Ht 63 in, Wt 200 lbs, BP 90/60 mmHg, HR 64/min, RR 14/min, Temp 98.2 F.

General Examination:

GENERAL APPEARANCE: obese, alert, well hydrated, in no distress.

HEAD: normocephalic, atraumatic.

EYES: pupils equal, round, reactive to light and accommodation, extraocular movement intact.

EARS: tympanic membrane intact, clear.

ORAL CAVITY: mucosa moist, good dentition.

THROAT: no erythema, no exudate.

NECK/THYROID: no cervical lymphadenopathy, no thyroid nodules, no thyromegaly.

SKIN: multiple small tattoos, warm and dry, normal hair distribution, no suspicious lesions.

HEART: S1, S2 normal, regular rate and rhythm, no murmurs, rubs, gallops, no clicks. LUNGS: clear to auscultation bilaterally.

ABDOMEN: bowel sounds present, soft, nontender, nondistended, no hepatosplenomegaly, no guarding or rigidity.

BACK: mild TTP LLB, full range of motion of trunk w/o pain, normal exam of spine, spine nontender to palpation, no costovertebral angle tenderness.

MUSCULOSKELETAL: guarding when attempt to check radial pulse right wrist, unable to perform ROM on right wrist d/t pain, mild TTP and ROM of left wrist and thumb, + MCP squeeze BL, no apparent synovitis or erythema. Cervical spine normal, full range of motion, full range of motion of the hip, lumbosacral spine normal. + MTP squeeze left foot, no pain on ROM of knees, ankles, no swelling or deformity.

EXTREMITIES: +1 pitting edema BL ankles, good capillary refill in nail beds, no clubbing, cyanosis.

PERIPHERAL PULSES: 2+ dorsalis pedis, 2+ posterior tibial, 2+ radial.

NEUROLOGIC: nonfocal, alert and oriented, cerebellar function normal, cognitive exam grossly normal, cooperative with exam, cranial nerves II–XII grossly intact, deep tendon reflexes 2+ symmetrical, gait normal, motor strength normal upper and lower extremities, neck supple, no rigidity, no tremor.

PODIATRIC: normal.

PSYCH: alert, oriented, cognitive function intact, cooperative with exam, good eye contact, judgment and insight good, speech clear, thought content without suicidal ideation, delusions.

Critical Thinking:

1) What are the major concerns in this case?
2) What is your plan for Ivanna?
3) What patient teaching is appropriate at this time?

Junior

HPI: Junior is a 73-year-old African male who reports right knee pain and swelling for four weeks. He is taking Tylenol, which has helped.

Medications:

Aspirin EC 81 mg delayed release 1 tablet once a day.
Sildenafil citrate 50 mg 1 tablet as needed ½ hour – 4 hours prior to sexual activity.
Hydrochlorothiazide 25 mg 1 tablet in the morning once a day.
Carvedilol 25 mg orally two times per day.
Amlodipine besylate 10 mg 1 tablet once a day.

Medical/Surgical History:

Hypertension.

FMH:

Parents: deceased, unknown causes.
Eight siblings: alive and well in home country.
Spouse and children are alive and well.

SH:

Denies use of tobacco, alcohol, or recreational drugs.
Living with spouse. Unemployed.
Junior was a government official who had to flee his home country.

Allergies: NKDA.

ROS:

General/constitutional: denies fever, chills.
HEENT: denies headaches. Reports visual problems but sees an eye doctor annually. Denies ear pain, problems with hearing, vertigo, tinnitus, nasal congestion, epistaxis. Needs dental screening and cleaning.

Cardiovascular/respiratory: denies chest pain, dizziness, palpitations, dyspnea. Admits to fluid accumulation in the legs and orthopnea.

GI/GU: reports hiccups at night. Admits to eating spicy food. Denies heartburn, but if he eats late, then he hiccups. Denies abdominal pain, blood in stool or urine, constipation, diarrhea, difficulty swallowing or urinating, nausea, vomiting.

Musculoskeletal: Junior reports that he took a long walk. Shortly after, his right knee started hurting. Two days later, he went to the hospital for an US. He was told he might have arthritis. The US was negative for a DVT. He was told to use RICE for comfort. He is using heat and ice.

Skin: Junior denies concerns about his hair, skin, or nails

Neurologic: denies balance difficult, dizziness, memory loss, tingling/numbness.

Psychiatric: denies anxiety or depression.

Vital Signs:

Ht 72 in, BP 140/86 mmHg, HR 72/min, RR 16/min, Temp 98.4 F.

General Examination:

GENERAL APPEARANCE: alert, well hydrated, in no distress, well developed, well nourished. Presents in wheelchair because his knee hurts.

HEAD: normocephalic, atraumatic.

EYES: pupils equal, round, reactive to light and accommodation, extraocular movement intact, fundus normal.

NECK/THYROID: no cervical lymphadenopathy, no jugular venous distention, no thyromegaly.

HEART: S1, S2 normal, regular rate and rhythm, no murmurs, rubs, gallops, no clicks.

LUNGS: clear to auscultation bilaterally.

MUSCULOSKELETAL: no swelling or deformity of either knee. He cannot extend right leg d/t pain. There is noticeable swelling of the medial malleolus RLE. He says he has had this for a long time.

EXTREMITIES: good capillary refill in nail beds.

PERIPHERAL PULSES: 2+ dorsalis pedis, 2+ posterior tibial, 2+ popliteal.

NEUROLOGIC: alert and oriented, cooperative with exam, cognitive exam grossly normal, deep tendon reflexes 2+ symmetrical, limited strength RLE.

Critical Thinking:

1) What are the major concerns in this case?

2) What is your plan for Junior?

3) What teaching is appropriate at this time?

11

Other

Julio

HPI: Julio, a 45-year-old Latino male, presents with a request for a lab order for a urine test from a doctor in his home country. He reports urinary burning for three months. He was seen here by another provider who examined his prostate and started him on tamsulosin. He was referred to urology but could not afford to go to a urologist in the United States. Instead, he consults a urologist in his home country by phone. The urologist put Julio on HCTZ 25 mg and allopurinol 300 mg to prevent kidney stones. Julio has a history of kidney stones. The urologist would like Julio to have a 24-hour urine test. Julio reports pain in his penis during urination and says tamsulosin does not help with dysuria. He also expresses concern about "a swollen area" in his anus. After he has a BM and wipes himself, the swelling "goes back inside" his body. He also reports pain in the lower abdomen with a lot of flatulence. He is not taking omeprazole prescribed previously. He says his appetite is normal.

Medications:

Allopurinol 300 mg 1 tablet orally once a day.
Hydrochlorothiazide 25 mg 1 tablet in the morning orally once a day.
Tamsulosin HCl 0.4 mg capsule extended release 1 orally once a day.

Caring for the Displaced and Uninsured: Clinical Case Studies in Nursing & Healthcare,
First Edition. Leslie Neal-Boylan.
© 2023 John Wiley & Sons Ltd. Published 2023 by John Wiley & Sons Ltd.

Medical/Surgical History:

Lower tract obstructive urinary symptoms.

Nephrolithiasis.

Surgical removal of kidney stone—right side.

FMH:

Mother: deceased, lung cancer.

Father: alive and well.

Two sons: alive and well.

SH:

Drinks six beers on each weekend day and occasionally uses marijuana.

Denies tobacco use.

Lives alone. Works full time as a floor installer.

Allergies: Pollen: sneezing, watery eyes.

Vital Signs:

Ht 67 in, Wt 157 lbs, BP 124/78 mmHg, HR 90/min, RR 16/min, Temp 98.2 F.

General Examination:

GENERAL APPEARANCE: alert, well hydrated, in no distress, shakes his legs up and down while sitting. Appears anxious.

EYES: pupils equal, round, reactive to light and accommodation.

SKIN: warm and dry.

HEART: S1, S2 normal, regular rate and rhythm, no murmurs, rubs, gallops, no clicks.

LUNGS: clear to auscultation bilaterally.

ABDOMEN: bowel sounds present, soft, nontender, nondistended, no hepatosplenomegaly, no guarding or rigidity.

RECTAL: multiple condyloma acuminatum around the anus. One external hemorrhoid. Prostate is slightly enlarged, no masses palpable, no melena, no red blood, stool guaiac negative.

EXTREMITIES: good capillary refill in nail beds, no clubbing, cyanosis, or edema.

PERIPHERAL PULSES: 2+ radial.
NEUROLOGIC: nonfocal, alert and oriented.

Critical Thinking:

1) What are the major concerns in this case?
2) What is your plan for Julio?
3) What teaching is appropriate at this time?

Mario

HPI: Mario, a 45-year-old male, is a new patient who never had a medical visit. He reports left-sided chest pain for five years. He is unaware of any pattern with food or hunger but admits to feeling acid and a "burning" sensation in his chest. He takes an OTC medication of unknown name that helps. Mario does not read or write. He also reports pain in his left leg from hip to foot and BL plantar pain.

Medication:

OTC medicine for acid reflux.

Medical/Surgical History:

None.

FMH:

Both parents are deceased; age at time of death and causes of death are unknown. Two brothers are alive and well. No spouse/partner or children.

SH:

Previous smoker of cigarettes from age 14 years until three years ago. Denies use of alcohol or recreational drugs. Lives in a friend's basement. Works full time at a restaurant as a bus boy.

Allergies: NKDA.

ROS:

General: denies chills, fever, fatigue.

HEENT: denies headaches, problems with vision, dental problems. Never had eye or dental exam.

Cardiovascular/respiratory: admits to chest pain left side of chest at rest and with exertion, with left axillary pain × five years. Pain is intermittent; it starts daily, early in the morning. He has more pain after eating. Denies fluid accumulation in the legs or palpitations. Denies cough, hemoptysis, pain with inspiration, shortness of breath at rest or with exertion.

GI/GU: admits to heartburn. Denies abdominal pain, blood in the stool or urine, change in bowel or bladder habits, constipation, diarrhea, nausea, vomiting.

Musculoskeletal: Mario reports LLE pain from his left hip to his left foot but mostly in left hip and knee. Describes the pain as "shooting," not burning or throbbing. He also reports BL foot pain, plantar surfaces. He wears special shoes for work. He lifts heavy things and bends a lot at work.

Skin: denies rash, itching, skin lesion(s).

Neurologic: denies tingling/numbness, dizziness, memory changes.

Psychiatric: denies anxiety, depressed mood.

Vital Signs:

Ht 66 in, Wt 160 lbs, BP 132/85 mmHg, HR 70/min, RR 16/min, Temp 97.8 F.

General Examination:

GENERAL APPEARANCE: alert, well hydrated, in no distress.

HEAD: normocephalic, atraumatic.

EYES: pupils equal, round, reactive to light and accommodation, extraocular movement intact.

ORAL CAVITY: mucosa moist, partial dentures—upper.

NECK/THYROID: no cervical lymphadenopathy, no jugular venous distention, no thyroid nodules, no thyromegaly.

SKIN: two scars on left cheek; otherwise, warm and dry, normal hair distribution, no suspicious lesions.

HEART: S1, S2 normal, regular rate and rhythm, no murmurs, rubs, gallops, no clicks.

LUNGS: clear to auscultation bilaterally.

ABDOMEN: bowel sounds present, soft, nontender, nondistended, no hepatosplenomegaly, no guarding or rigidity.

BACK: full range of motion, normal exam of spine, spine nontender to palpation.

MUSCULOSKELETAL: FROM of left hip and left knee with mild pain, no pain on ROM of left thigh or ankle. Negative SLR. Otherwise FROM w/o pain, no swelling or deformity, FROM of trunk w/o pain.

EXTREMITIES: good capillary refill in nail beds, no clubbing, cyanosis, or edema, full range of motion.

PERIPHERAL PULSES: 2+ dorsalis pedis, 2+ posterior tibial, 2+ radial.

NEUROLOGIC: nonfocal, alert and oriented, cerebellar function normal, cognitive exam grossly normal, cooperative with exam, CNs II–XII grossly intact, deep tendon reflexes 2+ symmetrical, motor strength normal upper and lower extremities, no rigidity, no tremor.

PSYCH: alert, oriented, cognitive function intact, cooperative with exam, good eye contact, judgment and insight good, speech clear, thought content without suicidal ideation, delusions.

Critical Thinking:

1) What are the major concerns in this case?
2) What is your plan for Mario?
3) What teaching is appropriate at this time?

Ramon

HPI: Ramon, a 25-year-old male, presents for a posthospital visit. He has not been to the clinic in three years. Ramon was brought to the ED by EMS for alcohol and cocaine intoxication. A CXR was negative; an abdominal US showed a mildly fatty liver. An MRI of the brain was negative. On discharge, his AST was 2340, ALT >3300, CPK 57,760. Ramon says he had been taking oxycodone prior to the hospitalization, as well as "PCP," Tylenol, penicillin, and "one beer" for a toothache. He obtained the medications from the Latin store. Ramon was diagnosed with acute hepatitis related to hypertension, rhabdomyolysis, Tylenol, and alcohol. He was discharged on thiamine 100 mg/day, folic acid 1 mg/day, lactulose 15 ml twice a day, and melatonin. Ramon denies current use of alcohol or any recreational drug. He says he is trying to drink a lot of water. He reports mild abdominal pain and wants his liver checked. He reports nausea and chills but denies fever, vomiting, diarrhea, or constipation. He is currently unemployed. He reports he is sleeping well with melatonin.

Medications:

Vitamin D (cholecalciferol) 25 mcg (1000 UT) 1 capsule orally once a day.
Lexapro 20 mg 1 tablet a day for 7 days, then increase to 2 tablets/day orally once a day.
Acetaminophen 325 mg 1 tablet as needed, every 4 hours.
Aspirin 325 mg 1 tablet once a day.
Naproxen 500 mg 1 tablet with food or milk as needed, every 12 hours.
Melatonin 5 mg at bedtime.
Thiamine 100 mg once daily.
Folic acid 1 mg daily.

Medical/Surgical History:

Acute hepatitis.
HTN.

FMH:

Parents: alive and well.
Siblings: alive and well.
No spouse/partner or children.

SH:

Ramon smokes 10 cigarettes/day "for as long as I can remember." Admits to 10 or more alcoholic drinks per day, typically beer. Admits to using PCP "but not cocaine." He is living with family. Uses condoms. Has sexual intercourse with women only. Denies STIs.

Vital Signs:

Ht 65 in, Wt 205 lbs, BP 118/60 mmHg, HR 62/min, RR 14/min, Temp 98.2 F.

General Examination:

GENERAL APPEARANCE: obese, alert, well hydrated, in no distress, multiple tattoos.

EYES: pupils equal, round, reactive to light and accommodation, extraocular movement intact.

ORAL CAVITY: mucosa moist, poor dentition.

NECK/THYROID: no cervical lymphadenopathy, no jugular venous distention, no thyroid nodules, no thyromegaly.

SKIN: warm and dry.

HEART: S1, S2 normal, regular rate and rhythm, no murmurs, rubs, gallops, no clicks.

LUNGS: clear to auscultation bilaterally.

ABDOMEN: bowel sounds present, soft, mild TTP RUQ and LLQ. No rebound, no hepatosplenomegaly, no guarding or rigidity.

EXTREMITIES: good capillary refill in nail beds, no clubbing, cyanosis, or edema.

PERIPHERAL PULSES: 2+ dorsalis pedis, 2+ posterior tibial, 2+ radial.

NEUROLOGIC: nonfocal, alert and oriented, no rigidity, no tremor, cognitive exam grossly normal, cooperative with exam, deep tendon reflexes 2+ symmetrical.

PSYCH: alert, oriented, cognitive function intact, cooperative with exam, good eye contact, judgment and insight good, speech clear, thought content without suicidal ideation, delusions.

Critical Thinking:

1) What are the major concerns in this case?
2) What is your plan for Ramon?
3) What teaching is appropriate at this time?

Part II

Dilemmas and Decisions

12

Family Issues

Evangeline

Critical Thinking:

1) What are the major concerns in this case?

DMT2; Evangeline has not taken any medication in six months.
She lives with her employer; her family is in the Philippines.
PMH of CVA.
LE edema.
She has diminished sensation in her feet.
Has not had preventive screening.
Dizziness.
Left hip and LB pain.
Stress.

2) What is your plan for Evangeline?

BW: CBC, CMP, HgBA1C, lipid panel, TSH, UA, FIT.
Give Evangeline clonidine 0.1 mg now and recheck BP.
Prescribe lisinopril tablet, 20 mg, 1 tablet, once a day.
Prescribe metformin 850 mg with breakfast and with dinner.
Prescribe chlorthalidone or HCTZ 25 mg daily.
Give Evangeline a note for her employer to be off work today and tomorrow.
Refer Evangeline for free vision and dental screening if she meets eligibility requirements.

Caring for the Displaced and Uninsured: Clinical Case Studies in Nursing & Healthcare, First Edition. Leslie Neal-Boylan.
© 2023 John Wiley & Sons Ltd. Published 2023 by John Wiley & Sons Ltd.

Schedule Evangeline for Pap smear, give her an order for a mammogram, refer her for a colonoscopy.

Recommend Tylenol prn for musculoskeletal pain. She may also alternate ice and heat.

Recommend Meclizine 12.5 mg, one to two tablets daily to relieve dizziness.

3) What teaching is appropriate at this time?

Evangeline is asked to record her BP at least one hour after taking her medicine and bring the BP record to the next visit. She is to avoid salt in her diet and elevate legs when sitting. She is asked to rest today and tomorrow. She is asked to increase her water intake.

Evangeline is given a glucometer and instructed how to use it. She is to record FBGs twice per week and two-hour postprandial BG once per week and bring the record to the next visit.

Teach Evangeline how to check her feet daily and to apply moisturizing cream to her feet.

Evangeline RTC in two weeks for FU:

HPI: Evangeline reports she is taking medicine as prescribed. FBGs average 180. Two-hour PP BG average 200. BPs average 130/84. She denies dizziness and is no longer taking meclizine.

Lab results:

CBC WNL.
CMP: calcium 14; glucose 293.
Hemoglobin A1c 12.0.
Microalbumin/creatinine ratio: WNL.
Cholesterol, total: 206; HDL: 51; triglycerides: 180; LDL: 123.
TSH: 1.220.
Urinalysis, routine WNL.

Evangeline's diabetes is uncontrolled. Metformin is increased to 1000 mg twice a day with food. An ionized calcium test is ordered. However, since the albumin is normal, the calcium is unlikely to be actually elevated.

Evangeline will continue to measure her blood sugars and monitor her diet. Her BG is likely to continue to be high, so glipizide will be added. If her next HbGA1C remains very high, the clinician will start her on insulin and stop the glipizide.

Evangeline should monitor her BP and bring the record to the next visit.

Atorvastatin 10 mg every evening is added to the regimen. Evangeline is given instructions for diabetic and low cholesterol diets.

Pearl: In addition to her health issues, Evangeline is in a difficult living situation. She is widowed and alone in this country. She is working to save money to rejoin her children in her home country. She lives with her employer, which is likely to add to her stress. The patient was not able to access some of the free screenings offered to patients who complete specific county health forms. While she was eligible for these resources, her employer refused to provide the necessary information as her landlord and employer. Newer diabetic drugs are too expensive for patients without insurance.

Florence

Critical Thinking:

1) What are the major concerns in this case?
   Trigger finger.
   Right elbow pain.
   Possible carpal tunnel syndrome.
   LBP.
   BL hip pain.
   Cleans houses for a living.
   Father, whom she has not seen for 14 years, died in home country.
2) What is your plan for Florence?
   Check BW: ESR, ANA, rheumatoid factor, CCP antibodies.
   Florence's finger was splinted. She was told to RTC in six weeks if there was no improvement for a steroid injection.
   Show a picture to Florence of splints that she can wear at night to help prevent numbness and tingling in the UEs.
   Florence cleans houses for a living, so she cannot avoid musculoskeletal traumas and strain. Supportive care is helpful.
   Suggest Florence use a heating pad or warm towel on back or hips to help relieve pain.
   Listening is the important tool during this visit with Florence, allowing her to cry and reminisce about her father. Offer bereavement counseling if available.
3) What is appropriate teaching at this time?
   Florence is taught how to care for her finger and when to wear the splint. The clinician explains what trigger finger is and how it develops. She is advised to take NSAIDs as needed. She is advised that if she

has a steroid injection it may not last and she may require surgery. She may want to discuss the financial implications with family members and put aside some money in case surgery is necessary.

> Pearl: The clinician is liberal with providing "rest from work" notes for patients who have very physical jobs to allow them to rest their joints. A CRP is not ordered to avoid unnecessary expense. EMG and nerve conduction studies are very expensive.

Gloria

Critical Thinking:

1) What are the major concerns in this case?
   Constipation.
   High carbohydrate diet.
   Grief r/t recent loss of mother in Africa.
   Obesity.
2) What is your plan for Gloria?
   Refer to behavioral health.
   Offer active listening.
3) What patient teaching is appropriate at this time?
   Take Metamucil daily. Take one large spoonful with a large glass of water. Increase water intake daily to 8–12 glasses. Increase exercise, fruit and vegetable intake.

> Pearl: Some foods are common to certain cultures. While not everyone eats the same foods, many people within a culture share common tastes. These foods may cause flatulence, acid reflux, distention, and abdominal pain. Teaching patients about the effects of these foods on their symptoms can frequently obviate the need for medications. It is important to help patients reduce carbohydrates in ways that will not interfere with eating the food with which they have grown up. Suggesting reduced amounts is helpful as is encouraging increased intake of fruits, vegetables, and water. It is not uncommon for African women to perceive their obesity as normal and beautiful. They may consider weight loss unnecessary and unhealthful.

13

Medication Issues

Ali

Critical Thinking:

1) What are the major concerns in this case?
   History of syncope.
   DMT2: does not check BG; lack of knowledge about DM.
   Hyperlipidemia: stopped taking medicine.
   Refuses women's health screenings.
   Osteoporosis.
   High blood pressure.
2) What is your plan for Ali?
   BW: hemoglobin A1c, CMP, vitamin D3.
   Refill insulin.
   Give Ali a glucometer and teach her how to use it and when to check her BG.
   Restart atorvastatin.
   Order DEXA scan.
   Start low-dose medicine for blood pressure and bring patient back in two weeks for CMP and BP check.
   Order FIT and colonoscopy for screening.

Caring for the Displaced and Uninsured: Clinical Case Studies in Nursing & Healthcare, First Edition. Leslie Neal-Boylan.
© 2023 John Wiley & Sons Ltd. Published 2023 by John Wiley & Sons Ltd.

Based on ASCVD guidelines, determine whether Ali should continue taking aspirin daily.

3) What teaching is appropriate at this time?

Explain what causes DMT2 and clarify questions. Explain the importance of avoiding hypoglycemic symptoms through diet management and taking insulin appropriately.

Instruct Ali to continue the insulin regimen as prescribed. She should avoid sugar and bread products. Ali should try to keep her FBG under 140 (between 95 and 120); she should check FBGs twice per week and check one BG two hours after the biggest meal. It's important to consider the acceptable range for blood sugar for each patient based on age and history of hypoglycemic symptoms. It's also important to consider culture related to food preferences. While a lower range for acceptable blood sugar may be preferable per guidelines, patients whose diets consist of an abundance of carbohydrates may be less compliant if the parameters are set too low.

Ali should record the numbers and bring the BG record to the next visit. Advise Ali to get ophthalmological exam annually. She should try to get an appointment with an endocrinologist who takes Medicaid.

Ali is encouraged to restart and continue atorvastatin every evening and eat a low-fat diet. She is told it is important to exercise daily and drink 8–12 glasses of water daily.

Ali is advised to pick a pharmacy and check her BP two to three times/week and record the numbers. She is instructed in the correct way to measure BP: feet flat on the floor, rest a full five minutes, elevate the arm to the level of her heart, and take the BP. She is asked to bring the record of top and bottom numbers and heart rate to the next visit. She is asked to avoid salt in her diet.

The clinician and Ali discuss importance of regular preventative screening.

Pearl: It is not unusual for patients to misunderstand how the body works. Frequently, provider instructions are misunderstood or misconstrued. This can happen to any patient from any culture or country regardless of educational background. It is important to explain the cause of the condition or disease to reassure the patient, make the person a partner in care, and encourage adherence to the plan of treatment.

Ethan

Critical Thinking:

1) What are the major concerns in this case?
   Ethan is nonadherent with a diabetic diet; he rarely checks his BG.
   He has peripheral neuropathy.
   He is a smoker.
   He drinks alcohol excessively.
   He works as an auto mechanic, exposing him to injury.
2) What is your plan for Ethan?
   BW: CBC, CMP, lipid panel, HgBA1C, albumin/creatinine ratio before the next visit.
   Ethan refuses a flu shot and a TDaP.
   Refill metformin HCL 1000 mg, 1 tablet with a meal, twice a day.
   Refill glipizide, 10 mg, 1 tablet 30 minutes before breakfast and dinner, twice a day.
   Refill atorvastatin calcium 20 mg, 1 tablet, once a day.
3) What teaching is appropriate at this time?
   Ethan refuses to start insulin. The clinician has a long talk with Ethan, via an interpreter, about the need to start insulin. Ethan admits he is afraid to start insulin because, in his view, his parents died after starting insulin and because he is afraid to inject himself. The clinician explains that Ethan's parents were probably experiencing serious complications by the time they started insulin, and then it was not the insulin that killed them. He responds that he will think about it.

   The clinician emphasizes that Ethan should avoid sugar, limit tortillas to one tortilla twice per week, change bread to low-sugar wheat bread, and eat only one or two slices per week. The use of the glucometer is reviewed. Ethan is advised to check his BG twice per week before breakfast and once per week two hours after any meal. He should vary the meals after which he checks his BG. Ethan is asked to record the results and bring them to the next visit. The clinician explains the need to tightly control the BG to avoid complications such as loss of vision or limbs or kidney failure. He is to check his feet daily for open wounds or calluses and use lotion to prevent dry skin on his feet. Ethan is reminded to return to the eye doctor next week for FU.

Ethan is reminded that smoking is detrimental to his health and that alcohol can damage his liver and cause chronic disease. The clinician offers to connect Ethan with support groups for people with alcohol use disorder. At the next visit, the clinician will offer a medicine to help him stop smoking.

Ethan RTC in three months for FU:

HPI: Ethan reports he is taking his medication as prescribed. He has only checked his BGs once. Yesterday, the FBG was 170 and the two-hour postprandial reading was 200. Ethan denies signs or symptoms of hypoglycemia but says the plantar surfaces of his feet "burn and sweat" at night. He admits that he has not modified his diet. He has cut down on cigarettes to three per day and has cut down his alcohol intake to six beers per day. He says he feels generally well today.

Results of BW:

CBC WNL.
CMP: elevated LFTs, elevated glucose.
Lipid panel: LDL is 160, HDL is 35.
Albumin: elevated.
HgBA1C: 11.0.

The clinician explains that uncontrolled DM is having serious effects on Ethan's kidneys, his cholesterol is abnormal, and his liver function is abnormal. Ethan admits that he does not take his atorvastatin daily. The clinician reinforces the likelihood of complications of uncontrolled DM and encourages Ethan to start insulin. She explains that insulin can help him avoid complications and death from DM, as occurred with his parents. Insulin will also give him a bit more flexibility in what he eats. Ethan agrees to start insulin. The clinician begins with Novolin N twice a day. The RN reviews use of the glucometer and BG testing and demonstrates how Ethan will draw up the medicine and administer it to himself. He is instructed regarding what to do if he has symptoms of hypoglycemia and to record his BGs regularly. The clinician will likely add Novolin R to the regimen at the next visit but recognizes that it is necessary to go slowly and not overwhelm Ethan.

Ethan is praised for reducing his tobacco and alcohol intake and encouraged to keep up the good work to continue to reduce his use.

> Pearl: There have been many recent developments in DM management and treatment. However, uninsured patients cannot afford newer medications. A basal insulin would be ideal for Ethan, but giving him Novolin N twice a day will give him similar coverage and is much less expensive. It would be helpful to have Ethan use CGM (continuous glucose monitoring) for 14 days. Although he has a cell phone to use as a sensor, the CGM is beyond his budget.

Juan

Critical Thinking:

1) What are the major concerns in this case?
   Juan has kidney stones that are painful.
   Juan cannot afford to see the urologist.
   Juan works as a landscaper; there are considerations related to his work. His work is very physical. He is exposed to hazardous sprays and insecticides.
   Juan has never had vision or dental exams.
   Juan is constipated.
   Juan has back pain.
   Juan took Amoxicillin without a prescription.
2) What is your plan for Juan?
   Renal or abdominal ultrasound.
   Treat Juan's pain.
   Ask clinic staff to see if Juan qualifies for any financial assistance so he can see a urologist.
   Refer Juan for free vision and dental screening.
   Give Juan a TDaP.
3) What patient teaching is appropriate at this time?
   Juan requires instruction regarding what kidney stones are, why they occur, and how to prevent them.
   Juan needs a tetanus shot if he hasn't had one in 10 years, particularly because he works in landscaping; he may need catch-up

vaccinations but the clinic cannot afford to stock all of the necessary vaccinations, and they are very expensive without insurance.

Juan should be instructed regarding why he should not take antibiotics without consulting his healthcare provider.

He should be instructed regarding a high-fiber diet and how to improve his nutrition. The provider will offer nutritional counseling, including a diet sheet in Spanish if Juan can read. The provider should also offer information regarding local food pantries and what constitutes a healthful diet.

Pearl: It is not uncommon for patients to get medications sent to them from their home country without a prescription or get them from a local Latin store. Also, it is expensive to get many of the vaccinations required in the United States; however, patients who work in construction or in landscaping are especially vulnerable to tetanus and should receive the vaccination.

Margarita

Critical Thinking:

1) What are the major concerns in this case?
   No previous medical visit or blood work.
   Right hip and LB pain.
   Recent fall.
   Headache.
   Strong family history of several chronic illnesses.
   Use of alternative remedies that may/may not be appropriate.
   Scars from cupping.
   Use of trazodone, a potentially habit-forming medicine.
2) What is your plan for Margarita?
   Find out more about Margarita's headaches by asking focused questions.
   Margarita requires a CPE and initial blood work; consider imaging right hip.
   Blood work for lipid panel, CMP, CBC, thyroid panel, UA, HgBA1C.
   Screening mammogram and Pap smear.
   FIT and/or colonoscopy.
   Margarita needs referral for free vision and dental screening.
   Margarita likely needs catch-up immunizations, but they are expensive.

Check orthostatic BPs to see if Margarita might be hypotensive.

PT might help Margarita, but it is costly. If imaging of right hip is negative for fracture but she continues to have pain, a CT scan is appropriate. If these are negative for fracture, give her written information in Spanish and have an interpreter explain how she can do some exercises to strengthen her hips and LB to alleviate and prevent pain.

Suggest alternating Tylenol and ibuprofen for pain relief. Margarita can also heat a towel under hot water and apply it to her hip and back for pain relief.

3) What patient teaching is appropriate at this time?

Margarita should be advised to discuss alternative remedies with the clinician before using them.

Margarita should be encouraged to get the COVID-19 vaccines and taught why she needs them.

Margarita should be encouraged to take calcium with vitamin D twice a day unless she is getting sufficient supplementation through food.

Ask Margarita to try melatonin or valerian root for sleep instead of trazodone. Discuss the cause of her difficulty sleeping and consider referral to behavioral health if needed. Margarita has a FMH of depression.

Margarita may have increased risk of falling related to taking trazodone.

Ask Margarita to monitor her BP at a local pharmacy two to three times/week and explain how to properly assess BP. She should bring the record to her follow-up visit.

Ask Margarita to keep a headache diary or have someone she knows help her with that. Bring the record to next visit.

Pearl: Patients often arrive in the United States with knowledge of home remedies they used in their home countries, or their family members or friends share suggestions regarding home remedies. Rarely are they harmful. In those cases, the patient should be permitted to continue them. However, if they interact with other medications or are potentially harmful, it is best to explain this to the patient. Being open to harmless home remedies engenders trust in the clinician and fosters confidence when the clinician tells the patient about other treatments that might work better.

Paula

Critical Thinking:

1) What are the major concerns in this case?
   Paula stopped all her medications.
   Productive cough, headache, facial pain, "fever," dyspnea for 15 days.
   HTN.
   Obesity.
   Acid reflux.
   Hyperlipidemia.
   Prediabetes.
   Constipation.
   Vitamin D deficiency.
2) What is your plan for Paula?
   Fluticasone OTC (cheaper than prescription).
   Stop taking Mucinex.
   Increase fluid intake.
   Restart all other medications.
   Recheck BW in three months.
   Pap smear and mammogram.
3) What teaching is appropriate at this time?
   Explain to Paula that she should not stop or change her medications without consulting the provider. Stopping medications can cause the return or worsening of her health conditions.
   Paula should restart her medications and check her BP two to three times per week and bring record to next visit.

Pearl: Patients frequently stop their medications when they feel sick and treat themselves with herbal remedies or those that are culturally familiar. There is a pervasive perception that the medications, regardless of what they are, will make the acute condition worse.

Rosa

Critical Thinking:

1) What are the major issues in this case?
   Rosa delayed medical treatment and purchased an antibiotic at the Latin store. Her finger is now infected.
   Rosa is out of her medicines.
   Rosa's FMH is unknown.
2) What is your plan for Rosa?
   Treat Rosa's infection with cephalexin. She is eligible for free medications in the clinic closet, and that is one that is in stock. A wound culture is too expensive for Rosa.
   Refill Rosa's medications.
3) What patient teaching is appropriate at this time?
   Help Rosa understand antibiotic resistance and the importance of treating infections with the correct medicine.
   Explain that Rosa should be careful to not run out of her medicine. She should call the clinic one week before she runs out so prescriptions can be sent to her pharmacy.

> Pearl: Patients frequently think they no longer need their medicines once the prescription has finished. They don't always realize they may have a refill or how to obtain the refill. They may stop the medicine and not call for more or for a follow-up appointment.

Santiago

Critical Thinking:

1) What are the major concerns in this case?
   DMT2 with sporadic metformin use for treatment.
   Gets metformin without a prescription from his country.
   Weight loss of 30 pounds in three years.
   Possible peripheral neuropathy.
   High blood pressure.
   Irregular heart rate.

2) What is your plan of treatment?

Start metformin HCL 500 MG, 1 tablet with a meal, daily.

BW: CBC with differential/platelet, CMP, hemoglobin A1c, lipid panel, albumin/creatinine ratio, UA.

Next visit: foot check and EKG.

Refer him to a dentist.

3) What should be included in patient teaching for Santiago?

Restart metformin 500 mg with breakfast for now. We will probably increase it once lab results are back. Stop eating sugar and reduce your intake of bread, rice, tortillas, and pasta.

Take Neurontin 100 mg at night for burning pain.

Record BPs at a local pharmacy two to three times a week and bring the record to the next visit.

Santiago RTC for FU in one week:

HPI: Santiago presents with continuing burning pain in L-S spine and left thigh. He feels burning pain when his clothes touch his leg. Neurontin 100 mg at night is not helping. He reports that the pain comes around from his lower back to his pelvis and left thigh. He reports episodes of dizziness, palpitations, and chest pressure when doing heavy or strenuous work or physical exercise. He also feels palpitations and fatigue. He denies dyspnea, pain with breathing, or edema. He denies any symptoms at rest or being awakened by symptoms.

Vital Signs:

BP 130/72 mmHg, HR 100/min, RR 16/min, Temp 98.2 F.

General Examination:

GENERAL APPEARANCE: alert, well hydrated, in no distress.

HEART: S1, S2 normal, regular rate and rhythm, no murmurs, rubs, gallops, no clicks. EKG: NSR with tachycardia.

LUNGS: clear to auscultation bilaterally.

MUSCULOSKELETAL: negative SLR BL, lumbosacral spine is normal, full range of motion of the hip, no swelling or deformity.

EXTREMITIES: good capillary refill in nail beds, no clubbing, cyanosis, or edema.

PERIPHERAL PULSES: 2+ dorsalis pedis, 2+ posterior tibial, 2+ radial.
NEUROLOGIC: nonfocal, alert and oriented.
Based on the BW results, metformin is increased to 500 mg twice a day.
Neurontin is increased to 300 mg, once a day, at night.
The clinician orders an MRI of the lumbar spine and sacrum without
contrast and a CT of the abdomen.
Santiago is started on metoprolol 25 mg, once a day for high blood pres-
sure and palpitations. He is referred to cardiology and is instructed to
go to the ED if he has chest pain or pressure, palpitations, or dizziness
that don't go away. He is told to drink 8–12 glasses of water daily.

Santiago RTC two weeks later:

HPI: Santiago cannot sleep due to burning discomfort in his lower back,
lower abdomen, and genitals. When he is not wearing clothing, he
does not have as much pain. He says he lost his job because he is walking and working slowly due to the pain. He is taking 300 mg gabapentin at night with no relief. He reports a decrease in palpitations with
metoprolol. He now denies chest pressure or pain. He has mild dizziness when lifting heavy things at work. He reports he is eating well but
does not drink much water.

General Examination:

GENERAL APPEARANCE: alert, well hydrated, in no distress, appears
tired and somewhat frail.
EYES: pupils equal, round, reactive to light and accommodation, extraoc-
ular movement intact.
SKIN: warm and dry.
HEART: S1, S2 normal, regular rate and rhythm, no murmurs, rubs, gal-
lops, no clicks.
LUNGS: clear to auscultation bilaterally.
MUSCULOSKELETAL: no swelling or deformity, steady gait.
EXTREMITIES: good capillary refill in nail beds, no clubbing, cyanosis,
or edema.
PERIPHERAL PULSES: 2+ dorsalis pedis, 2+ posterior tibial, 2+ radial.
NEUROLOGIC: nonfocal, alert and oriented.
MRI of lumbar spine and sacrum showed a possible cyst or tumor of
nerves in the left pelvic wall and tendinopathy bilaterally in the lower

extremities, specifically, the hamstrings. An MRI of the left hip is recommended.

The CT scan of the abdomen is negative.

Following a phone call during which Santiago reports two episodes of near fainting and dizziness, the clinician refers him to neurology.

The MRI of the left hip shows a complex labral tear and mild OA.

The neurologist orders an MRI of the cervical spine that shows mild cervical disc protrusions at multiple levels.

The cardiologist continues metoprolol succinate ER 25 mg daily. A repeat EKG shows PVCs but is otherwise normal.

Pearl: Patients sometimes take their medications sporadically due to inability to pay for medication. Santiago was given a thorough workup to explore his health concerns. Each workup, including the specialty visits, imaging, and additional BW, ordered by the specialists, was costly. In addition, he lost his job due to his symptoms. Santiago was lost to follow-up.

14

Food or Housing Issues

Carmen

Critical Thinking:

1) What are the major concerns in this case?
   Cannot afford food.
   Hyperlipidemia.
   Vitamin D deficiency.
   Hypothyroidism.
   Palpitations.
   Weakness.
   FMH of alcoholism.
2) What is your plan for Carmen?
   BW: lipid panel, HgBA1C, TSH, T4, T3, vitamin D, CMP, CBC.
   Refill atorvastatin calcium, 40 mg, 1 tablet, once a day.
   Refill vitamin D3, 2000 unit, 1 capsule, daily.
   Refill levothyroxine sodium 75 mcg, 1 tablet in the morning on an empty stomach.
   Mammogram.
3) What patient teaching is appropriate at this time?
   Give Carmen information about local food banks. Provide oral and written information (if she can read) about a low-cholesterol diet.
   Advise Carmen to take calcium with vitamin D two to three times per week, depending on how much calcium she gets in her diet.

Caring for the Displaced and Uninsured: Clinical Case Studies in Nursing & Healthcare, First Edition. Leslie Neal-Boylan.
© 2023 John Wiley & Sons Ltd. Published 2023 by John Wiley & Sons Ltd.

Continue levothyroxine every morning ½ hour before eating or taking other medications.

Educate Carmen about her increased risk of alcoholism; the clinician offers to provide support if she needs it in the future.

Carmen presents for FU and review of BW:

HPI: Carmen states she is eating more meat and feels less weak but has been unable to access the food bank due to lack of transportation. She denies palpitations or epigastric pain. She has not yet received COVID-19 vaccinations. Carmen is anxious about her health and her living arrangements. She says she has enough food "sometimes."

Carmen is referred to a food bank that delivers food. She needs financial help to afford her medications. She is referred to the county's emergency assistance program. She is educated about the need to get COVID-19 vaccines and is encouraged to get free COVID-19 vaccines the clinic offers every Saturday. The clinic can help with transportation to get the vaccines. She is also referred to behavioral health.

> Pearl: Patients may not always reveal that they don't have access to food or healthful food. It is important to ask and offer information about local food banks. However, patients may not have transportation to food banks. Some offer food delivery service. Offer patients coupons to help them afford their medicine.

Luciana

Critical Thinking:

1) What are the major concerns in this case?

Luciana had to take several buses and walk two miles to reach the clinic.

She perceived discrimination when trying to find a place to live.

She cannot afford a lawyer to assist her.

Previous history of colon cancer.

Questionable mental health.

High blood pressure.

LLE pain.

2) What is your plan for Luciana?

Refer Luciana to emergency assistance if it is available in her area. Personnel can assist her with housing and legal representation.

Try to use clinic funds allotted to send Luciana home (to a friend's house) in a taxi or Uber car.

Refer Luciana to behavioral health if available at low cost.

Obtain FIT and/or refer for colonoscopy.

3) What teaching is appropriate at this time?

Explain that there is not currently sufficient evidence or rationale for getting x-rays or sending Luciana to a neurologist.

The clinician explains to Luciana that the clinic and county have resources that might help her; however, she must keep scheduled appointments. It is important she maintain her health with preventive screenings.

Ask Luciana to monitor her blood pressure at a local pharmacy two to three times a week and bring the record to the next visit. Advise Luciana to avoid salt in her diet.

> **Pearl:** Accessing transportation can be challenging for low-income patients. It is ideal if the clinic is located near a bus or subway line so patients are only required to walk short distances. The clinic should have some ad hoc funds to assist patients who need transportation but have mobility difficulties.

Michelle

Critical Thinking:

1) What are the major concerns in this case?

Michelle is homeless and unemployed; she is living in a shelter with two young children.

She has an abusive husband of whom she is afraid.

She has a uterine prolapse that requires surgical intervention.

She has no friends here.

She is due for a Pap smear.

2) What is your plan for Michelle?

It is important to spend time with Michelle to obtain her trust and reassure her that the clinic can help her. She is already connected with adult and child protective services.

If Michelle desires it, the clinician can offer to connect with her case managers.

Michelle needs a thorough pelvic exam with Pap smear. The clinician should be mindful of and sensitive to Michelle's history of abuse.

Michelle will need a referral to GYN for surgery. The clinician decides to send her to a local Catholic hospital because she will receive care at a lower cost. However, she will need to wait several months for an appointment. The clinician consults with a GYN colleague who contacts her colleague at the Catholic hospital. That GYN agrees to see the patient soon at a reduced cost.

The clinician refers Michelle to behavioral health and will collaborate with the therapist regarding whether Michelle will benefit from an antidepressant medication.

Michelle needs standard BW, such as: CBC, CMP, hemoglobin A1C, lipids, UA, TSH.

3) What patient teaching is appropriate at this time?

Instruct Michelle that the clinic is a resource and that the clinic can tap into other local resources to help her and her children.

Remind Michelle to call the police/911 if she is threatened by her husband.

Explain to Michelle that surgery will be costly but the clinic can help her apply for programs to get financial assistance.

Advise Michelle to go to Planned Parenthood for a pessary until she can see the GYN.

Pearl: Specialist colleagues who are willing to consult by phone with the clinician are vital to the primary care provider caring for the uninsured. They can be hugely helpful with guidance regarding assessment and treatment and frequently have their own colleagues who may be willing to see the patient at a reduced cost. Patients living in homeless shelters are subjected to fears regarding their safety, security of their possessions, cleanliness and hygiene, and access to resources. These patients may despair that they will ever leave the shelter. Single patients may be housed with roommates they don't know or trust.

Paul

Critical Thinking:

1) What are the major concerns in this case?

   Poor diet that has led to obesity.

   Uncontrolled DMT2; he does not check his BG.

   Paul is not taking his medicine.

   He gets medicine from his home country.

   He has not had a medical visit for two years.

   Smoker of tobacco and marijuana.

   Alcohol use disorder.

   Constipation and intermittent abdominal pain; acid reflux.

   Living situation.

   Paul has never had dental or vision screening.

   LE edema.

   Stressed d/t living situation and missing family in his home country.

   HBP.

   Uses bleach to resolve pruritic rash.

2) What is your plan for Paul?

   Refill Novolin 70/30. The clinician should start Paul with lower doses than he was taking two years ago and then increase as needed based on BG levels.

   Restart metformin 1000 mg twice a day with food.

   Do not restart glipizide given the risk of hypoglycemia when combined with insulin. Refer Paul to endocrinology, but it is likely to take several weeks to months to get an appointment.

   Refer for free vision and dental screenings.

   Conduct a diabetic foot exam next visit.

   Begin a low-dose ACEI for renal protection.

   Consider testing vitamin B12. Patient has been on metformin for a long time.

   Refill rosuvastatin 20 mg/day in the evening.

   Consider pulmonary CT scan due to Paul's history of smoking.

3) What patient teaching is appropriate at this time?

   Give Paul a free glucometer and remind him how and when to use it. He should check his fasting blood sugar twice/week and two-hour postprandial blood sugar once a week after any meal. He should try to vary the meals. He should bring a record of his BGs to his next visit.

Reinforce the need to eat a low-fat diet. Explain the Mediterranean or DASH diets and give Paul written information if he can read.

Discuss the importance of weight loss. Reinforce that fried and fast foods are high in fat and salt. Lemonade is high in sugar and acid. He should not add salt to food and should avoid foods that contain sodium or salt. He should be encouraged to walk 30 minutes/day. He should avoid sugar and limit intake of carbohydrates. Explain that alcohol turns to fat in the body. He should be encouraged to increase his intake of vegetables and low-sugar fruit such as some berries. Offer information about local food banks. Explain that fried and acidic foods in addition to heavy meals can contribute to abdominal pain and acid reflux. Paul does not have much money and is dependent on others for housing. He works making deliveries so fast food is a cheap and convenient way to get his meals. A discussion about diet will need to be ongoing. Paul will need support to change his diet and improve his overall health.

Discuss smoking and alcohol and help Paul understand why they are detrimental to his health. He returned to the clinic after two years; his DM is the priority at this time. However, it will be important to follow up with him about his smoking and drinking and offer resources for support. Many patients choose to quit or cut down on their own because smoking cessation remedies, including those that are OTC, can be expensive. Paul might be willing to go to Alcoholics Anonymous if there is a meeting near him.

Ask Paul to check his BP at a local pharmacy or grocery store twice a week, if possible, and bring the record to the next visit.

Explain that bleach can be absorbed into the blood stream and poison the blood. He can use Benadryl cream for a rash; however, he should RTC if the pruritic rash returns.

Paul RTC for FU in six months:

HPI: Paul went to his home country to visit his mother. He has not had any medicine for at least three months. He did not seek medical help in his country because COVID-19 is rampant there and the death rate is very high. He has not been checking his blood sugar. He denies signs or symptoms of hypoglycemia. He was taking insulin, metformin, and rosuvastatin as prescribed.

General Examination:

GENERAL APPEARANCE: obese, alert, well hydrated, in no distress.

EYES: pupils equal, round, reactive to light and accommodation, extraocular movement intact.

ORAL CAVITY: mucosa moist, some missing teeth.

NECK/THYROID: no cervical lymphadenopathy, no jugular venous distention, no thyroid nodules, no thyromegaly.

SKIN: warm and dry, brown papules along medial and ventral left wrist. Dry skin.

HEART: S1, S2 normal, regular rate and rhythm, no murmurs, rubs, gallops, no clicks.

LUNGS: clear to auscultation bilaterally.

ABDOMEN: obese, bowel sounds present, soft, nontender, nondistended, no hepatosplenomegaly, no guarding or rigidity.

BACK: no costovertebral angle tenderness, normal exam of spine, spine nontender to palpation, full range of motion.

MUSCULOSKELETAL: cervical spine normal, full range of motion, full range of motion of the hip, lumbosacral spine normal, no swelling or deformity.

EXTREMITIES: good capillary refill in nail beds, no clubbing, cyanosis, or edema.

PERIPHERAL PULSES: 2+ dorsalis pedis, 2+ posterior tibial, 2+ radial.

NEUROLOGIC: nonfocal, alert and oriented, cerebellar function normal, cognitive exam grossly normal, cooperative with exam, deep tendon reflexes 2+ symmetrical, motor strength normal upper and lower extremities, neck supple, no rigidity, no tremor.

PSYCH: alert, oriented, cognitive function intact, cooperative with exam, good eye contact, judgment and insight good, speech clear, thought content without suicidal ideation, delusions.

FOOT EXAM: sensory testing performed: sensations diminished. Sensory and motor testing performed: strength normal. Pedal pulse taking performed: 2+. Onychomycosis. Right great toe mildly erythematous, without swelling, warmth, or TTP.

New lab work is ordered: HgbA1C; CMP.

Paul is praised for walking daily and moderating his diet. His medications are refilled. He is now taking lisinopril 10 mg daily for renal protection and HTN. The education provided during the last visit is repeated. Paul is given clotrimazole cream, 1%, to apply to his irritated skin, twice a day. He is referred to a podiatrist and given a flu shot.

Pearl: Some patients are dependent on friends or family for housing. This fosters instability and makes adjustment to the United States more challenging. It also impacts transportation and access to food. Many uninsured patients, particularly immigrants, work in jobs related to food service. It may be kitchen work, restaurant service, food delivery, or housekeeping/cooking. Patients are likely to get their food at work; however, the food is not always consistent with their dietary needs. Patients may have difficulty transporting their own food to work, purchasing it, or making it at home to take to work. They may also feel stigmatized if they bring food to work when others are eating the food offered by employers. Those who eat at work may need to eat fast or on the run. The consequences are frequently acid reflux, excessive belching or flatulence, and abdominal pain.

15

Financial Issues

Glenda

Critical Thinking:

1) What are the major concerns in this case?
   Glenda experiences nightly asthma attacks.
   She takes Advair occasionally due to the high cost.
   Using either albuterol or Ventolin nightly.
   Perception of different care/treatment in ED because she is uninsured.
   Glasses broke and she cannot afford to fix them.
   Cavities and pain in teeth.
   Never had vision or dental exams.
   Unknown parental health history.
   Headaches related to stress; anxiety.
   Abdominal pain related to acid reflux.
   Obesity.
   Right knee pain.
   Left hip pain.
   LBP.
   Physically demanding job.
   DMT2; unable to tolerate metformin; cannot afford insulin if needed.
   Dyspnea at night.
   LE edema.
   Experienced many years of secondhand smoke.
   Stress UI and urgency; nocturia ×2.

Caring for the Displaced and Uninsured: Clinical Case Studies in Nursing & Healthcare, First Edition. Leslie Neal-Boylan.
© 2023 John Wiley & Sons Ltd. Published 2023 by John Wiley & Sons Ltd.

HTN.

Refuses x-ray due to cost.

2) What is your plan for Glenda?

Glenda needs an asthma plan that will work for her and that is affordable. The clinic cannot afford pulmonary function testing. Glenda is already taking montelukast. She should be encouraged to use Advair daily as prescribed. Once she runs out of it, prednisone might be added to her regimen. It is cheaper than most other drugs for asthma.

Glenda will be referred for free vision and dental screening.

The clinic might have grant money to help replace her glasses. Sometimes the county within a state has a program that can help.

Glenda has comorbidities that increase her risk of health problems, and her parental health history is unknown. She should be closely monitored with regular visits and blood work.

The clinician should explore Glenda's headaches in detail and consider referring to behavioral health, if available, for counseling.

Order CXR and musculoskeletal x-rays if Glenda is willing and able to afford them.

Consider adding HCTZ 12.5 mg or chlorthalidone daily to the medication regimen to reduce edema and BP. Wait until the patient brings back her BP record.

Glenda is a home health aide so her immunizations are probably UTD. Next visit, review preventative screening and order screening as needed.

3) What teaching is appropriate at this time?

Glenda should be encouraged to keep a diary of when she feels chest tightness, wheezing, coughing, or dyspnea; when she uses albuterol or Ventolin; and whether she gets relief. Explain Ventolin is albuterol.

Glenda experienced a disparity of care when she went to the ED. She should be encouraged to still go to the ED if her medicines are not working sufficiently to help her breathe.

Ask Glenda to limit salt in diet and elevate legs while sitting to reduce edema.

Ask Glenda to check and record her BP at a local pharmacy two to three times a week. Bring record to next visit.

Ask Glenda to check and record FBGs two times per week and a two-hour postprandial BG once per week and record these numbers. If possible, give her a free glucometer, strips, and lancets. Glenda may need to start insulin at the next visit since she cannot tolerate metformin. Newer drugs are too expensive.

Instruct Glenda regarding Kegel exercises and the role of obesity in urinary incontinence.

Explain that she probably has osteoarthritis and discuss possible treatments, such as applying heat, increasing exercise especially walking daily, and weight loss. She can take Tylenol for severe pain.

> Pearl: The clinician working with uninsured patients should always explore low-cost options regarding medications, procedures, and referrals. Advair and many other asthma medications are expensive. If the patient is given medications during a hospital stay or urgent care visit and has some medication remaining, then continue with that but have a backup plan ready to substitute that expensive medication with an affordable one. Equipment such as spirometry is expensive so may not be available in a clinic that subsists primarily on grant funding.

Guillermo

Critical Thinking:

1) What are the major concerns in this case?
   Guillermo has not been treated because he cannot afford treatment.
   He cannot work due to health issues.
   Abdominal discomfort with dizziness, nausea, and constipation.
   Anal itching.
   Knee pain.
   HBP.
2) What is your plan for Guillermo?
   BW: CBC, CMP, HgBA1C, lipid panel, UA.
   Stool for *H. Pylori*.
   Since Guillermo says he was diagnosed twice with *H. Pylori*, start treatment, but ask him to get the stool test before he starts taking the medication.
   Start Anusol cream for anal itching.
   Start omeprazole 20 mg daily

3) What patient teaching is appropriate at this time?

Avoid coffee, soda, spicy or fried foods, large meals, "fast food," and alcohol.

Advise Guillermo he can take Tylenol for knee pain and use heat but should not use NSAIDs.

Advise Guillermo to use baby wipes with glycerin to gently wipe his anus after toileting.

Guillermo RTC in two weeks for FU. The stool test was positive for *H. Pylori*:

HPI: Guillermo completed the 14-day course of medication for *H. Pylori*. He continues to have occasional abdominal pain but only when he eats late at night and then goes to sleep. He admits to drinking coffee and eating chili and other spicy foods late at night.

Guillermo is advised to continue taking omeprazole 20 mg daily. He is instructed to avoid coffee, spicy and fried foods, and heavy meals. He is asked to sit up for at least 30 minutes after eating.

Guillermo RTC in two months:

HPI: He reports difficulty sleeping for two months. He reports sleeping four to five hours and then being awakened by abdominal pain. He did not have this pain while taking omeprazole, but he ran out of the medicine. He says he has reduced his intake of spicy food and coffee. He is not drinking soda and has increased his water intake. He admits to eating a lot of beans and having mild nausea afterward. He denies vomiting, constipation, diarrhea, blood in the stool.

The previous instructions are reviewed with Guillermo. He is also asked to reduce gas-producing foods such as beans, cauliflower, broccoli, and acidic foods. He is told to take omeprazole ½ hour before eating dinner and to take two tablets of simethicone after dinner. Dicyclomine 20 mg 3 ×/day is prescribed prn abdominal pain.

Guillermo did not understand all instructions during the initial visit. He is also accustomed to eating certain foods. Repetition of instructions and assistance to make permanent dietary changes were necessary to resolve his symptoms. At a later visit, he reported he no longer needed dicyclomine or simethicone. He was taking omeprazole occasionally. He had lost some weight and felt much better.

> Pearl: Patients may not obtain necessary treatment because they cannot afford it and are unaware there are clinics or programs that can help. In this case, the patient lost his job as well, further limiting his financial means.

Lisette

Critical Thinking:

1) What are the major concerns in this case?
   Cellulitis of left leg.
   Possible DVT.
   DMT2.
   Delayed screening.
   Finances are a barrier to necessary care.
   Out of medicine.
   Takes medicine improperly.
   Alcohol use disorder.
   HTN.
   Overweight.
2) What is your plan for Lisette?
   Start cephalexin 500 mg, 1 tablet, four times a day, five days.
   BW: CBC, HgBA1C, CMP, lipid panel, UA, FIT (followed by colonoscopy).
   US: Doppler left leg.
   Refill aspirin 81 delayed release, 1 tablet, once a day- Plan to revisit the necessity of this once the current crisis is resolved.
   Refill metformin 1000 mg tablet, daily.
   Refill glipizide 5 mg tablet, once a day prebreakfast.
   Refill atorvastatin, 40 mg, once daily.
   Order a mammogram at the next visit.
3) What patient teaching is appropriate at this time?
   Take cephalexin 500 mg every six hours. (The clinic has cephalexin samples so she can start the antibiotic right away.) The clinician speaks to the patient and her granddaughter in the clinic and then speaks to the patient's daughter by phone. She explains the necessity of intravenous antibiotics and recommends going to the ED. The daughter reports the patient has no money and prefers to

first try the antibiotic by mouth. She says she will take Lisette to the ED tomorrow if there has been no improvement. The clinician explains that if there is any increase in redness or swelling or if either move up the leg, to take Lisette to the ED immediately. Lisette (via the granddaughter translating) and daughter (English-speaking) verbalize understanding of this plan. The clinician asks the patient to rest at home and to keep the leg elevated. She emphasizes the importance of getting the US today to rule out a DVT.

The clinician calls the patient 24 hours after this visit and speaks with the daughter, who speaks English:

The patient's daughter reports the swelling has decreased but the redness has not. Lisette says she had a lot of pain in the leg the previous night; she used ice and elevated the leg. She reports the leg is still swollen, but the pain has decreased. She says she has a blackened area on the leg that is "growing." The clinician tells Lisette and her daughter she must go to the ED immediately.

Pearl: This case illustrates how potentially dangerous it is when patients cannot access necessary care because of financial limitations. Lisette was told by the hospitalist that she had a high likelihood of dying from sepsis if she had waited any longer to go to the hospital. Clinicians in a clinic for the uninsured can use all resources (typically few in number and type) at their disposal; however, there are times when the patient must see a specialist or be hospitalized. Finances should not be a barrier to care. Lisette is responsible for some issues that have created barriers to care, such as her alcohol use disorder, her absence from the clinic for two years, and mismanagement of her medication. However, from her perspective, telehealth with her provider in another state was an acceptable way of continuing her care. The provider in the other state might have presumed the patient had no other access to care or assumed the patient was still living in that state. Patients who are immigrants frequently go back to their home countries for visits or go to other states where they have family and stay temporarily. It can also be difficult to get clinical notes and lab results from a patient's hospitalization. Some online programs can assist with this. Sometimes patients bring discharge notes with them, but they are frequently incomplete. Then, the continuum of care becomes additionally challenging.

Lisette RTC for follow-up three days later:

HPI: She presents for a posthospital FU for cellulitis. She was admitted to the hospital and treated with intravenous doxycycline and Augmentin. The Doppler was done at the hospital and was negative for DVT. She was also negative for osteomyelitis. Lisette reports the pain and swelling have decreased. She says she thinks she originally opened the skin on her leg because she often feels itchy; when she scratches, she opens the skin. She thinks that is cause of the cellulitis. She reports one reddened area remaining, smaller than previously, and burning pain on the plantar surfaces of her feet. She does not check BGs and does not know what they were in the hospital. She does not have a glucometer. She does not check her BP.

Vital Signs:

Wt 148 lbs, BP 162/88 mmHg, HR 76/min, RR 16/min, Temp 97.6 F, glucose 200, two hours after lunch.

General Examination:

GENERAL APPEARANCE: alert, well hydrated, in no distress.
EYES: pupils equal, round, reactive to light and accommodation.
SKIN: no edema or swelling of either LE. Mild erythema remains on anterior left ankle but is much improved. There are no open areas, lesions, or ulcers. The left medial ankle has ~0.5 cm patch of erythema, no open area, no edema/swelling/streaking. Both LEs are warm and dry.
HEART: S1, S2 normal, regular rate and rhythm, no murmurs, rubs, gallops, no clicks.
LUNGS: clear to auscultation bilaterally.
PERIPHERAL PULSES: 2+ dorsalis pedis, 2+ posterior tibial, 2+ radial.
NEUROLOGIC: nonfocal, alert and oriented.
HgBA1C: 7.6; CMP: elevated LFTs; CBC WNL; lipids: LDL 160, HDL 35; FIT is negative; UA WNL.

Critical Thinking:

1) What are the major concerns in this case?
   Cellulitis.
   DMT2.
   Alcohol use disorder.
   HTN.

Overweight.

Delayed screening.

Pruritis.

Hyperlipidemia.

Delayed screening

2) What is your plan for Lisette?

Start lisinopril tablet, 10 mg, 1 tablet, orally, once a day.

Continue metformin 1000 mg but increase it to twice daily with food.

Continue glipizide once daily.

Recheck HgBA1C and CMP in three months.

Offer Lisette affordable resources to help her cut down on alcohol use.

Order a mammogram.

Ask Lisette to RTC for a Pap smear.

Recommend Lisette get TDaP, pneumonia, and shingles vaccines.

3) What patient teaching is appropriate at this time?

The clinician asks Lisette to elevate her leg when sitting and to not scratch. She should complete the course of antibiotics.

Lisette should check and record her BP twice per week at a local pharmacy and bring the record to the next visit.

The clinician explains it is important to keep DM under control to avoid future infections. Lisette should check her feet daily and apply petroleum jelly to the skin on her arms, legs, and feet. She should use baby detergent and plain Dove soap for washing to avoid itching. Lisette should drink 8–12 glasses of water daily. The clinician advises Lisette to purchase a glucometer and check FBGs twice per week and two-hour postprandial BG once per week; bring the record to the next visit. She should continue taking metformin and glipizide daily and avoid sugar in her diet.

Lisette should continue taking atorvastatin every evening.

Explain the consequences of excessive alcohol intake and advise her to reduce her intake for her overall health. Recommend Alcoholics Anonymous.

Advise Lisette to get her medical care through one clinic where she can be seen in in person and occasionally via telehealth instead of getting medical care through a provider in another state.

Discuss the benefits of exercise and weight loss on HTN, DM, and cholesterol. Provide resources and teaching for good nutrition.

The clinician suggests Lisette try Benadryl at night for the itching and to use petroleum jelly or other OTC cream on skin.

Lisette's case was also complicated by the need for the clinician to talk to the patient through a teenaged granddaughter and then talk with the patient's daughter. While the clinic may rely on translators, frequently they are volunteers and are not always available, or the interpreter phone line is busy for a prolonged period, or the patient is simply more comfortable speaking with someone known and trusted. Another concern is compliance with HIPAA. Lisette was able to give her consent in person to her granddaughter and by phone to her daughter to speak with the clinician, but it is sometimes necessary to speak to a family member before the patient has had a chance to sign a HIPAA consent form. In these cases, it is necessary to have the patient give verbal consent, document that, and follow it up with a request for the consent in writing.

Lucia

Critical Thinking:

1) What are the major concerns in this case?

Deafness only partially alleviated with hearing aids; no affordable or accessible county or state resources.

Postoperative RUQ abdominal pain.

Financial concerns—paying hospital bills.

Occasional depression and PMH of suicide attempt.

Alcohol use disorder.

FMH of DM.

PMH of hepatitis B.

2) What is your plan for Lucia?

Refer Lucia to the county emergency assistance program for financial assistance.

Offer behavioral health referral.

Plan to assist Lucia to reduce alcohol intake.

Pap smear and discussion about birth control.

BW: CMP, lipid panel, CBC, HgBA1C, UA unless results from the recent surgery are available.

3) What teaching is appropriate at this time?

Lucia should avoid Tylenol. She can take ibuprofen but is discouraged from taking medication unless she has a lot of pain.

She is instructed that a heating pad or warm towel may provide comfort.

Lucia is instructed that reducing her alcohol intake will improve her overall health and help prevent liver damage and other chronic disease. Information about local groups is offered, but these are too expensive for Lucia at this time.

Lucia has not been introduced nor has she had access to resources for the deaf. These should be provided and assistance given to finance access if necessary or possible. Lucia is living in her mother's basement and is alone. She is unemployed and depressed with a history of a suicidal attempt. She will require close FU; the clinician should periodically check in with the behavioral health counselor.

Pearl: Resources for the deaf, hearing impaired, blind, and visually impaired may vary across counties and states. It can take months to get patients into free vision or dental screenings, and hearing aids may not be affordable. Basic vision screenings are possible at places like Costco and Walmart at a reduced cost. Eyeglasses may also be obtained at a reduced cost. It is important to be aware of resources in the area and to develop relationships with audiologists, EENTs, ophthalmologists, and dentists to try to negotiate reduced costs.

16

Work-Related Issues

Karla

Critical Thinking:

1) What are the major concerns in this case?
   Pain in right elbow.
   Numbness and tingling in BL wrists and hands.
   Lower back pain.
   BL hip pain.
   Irregular menses.
   Unknown parental medical history.
   New diagnosis of DMT2.
   Sero-negative RA?
   Hyperlipidemia.
   Widowed with three children.
   Depression and anxiety.
   PMH of STI.
2) What is your plan for Karla?
   If possible, send Karla to a rheumatologist. In any case, get lab work to possibly start methotrexate and folic acid: QuantiFERON Gold for TB, hepatitis B and C. Karla already had a CBC and a CMP. These two tests will be required every three months if Karla starts medication for RA. Start calcium with vitamin D daily.
   For now, Karla can start a trial of prednisone 20 mg daily for three days followed by 10 mg daily for three days. Refill atorvastatin.

Caring for the Displaced and Uninsured: Clinical Case Studies in Nursing & Healthcare, First Edition. Leslie Neal-Boylan.
© 2023 John Wiley & Sons Ltd. Published 2023 by John Wiley & Sons Ltd.

Offer behavioral health for depression. Ensure Karla feels safe in her environment.

Consider ordering an EMG and nerve conduction studies; however, these will be expensive.

Order pelvic ultrasound.

Start Karla on metformin 500 mg once a day with food.

Monitor Karla for chronic illnesses, given she has no knowledge of her parental medical history.

3) What patient teaching is appropriate at this time?

Suggest Karla try wetting a towel or wash cloth in hot water and applying to painful joints. She should be careful not to burn herself. If affordable, Karla can purchase a machine that melts wax and dip her hands and wrists when she has pain.

Show Karla a picture of CTS braces to purchase and wear at night. Avoid repetitive motion with arms, hands (this will be difficult since Karla is a painter). Offer a note to miss work for a few days. She should avoid sleeping on her arms.

Discuss low-fat and diabetic diets. Provide written diet sheets if Karla can read. Encourage exercise and weight loss.

Explain what diabetes is and why it is important to control it. Give Karla a free glucometer and teach her to check her FBG twice a week and her two-hour postprandial BG once a week, record the numbers, and bring record to the next visit.

Ensure Karla is able to obtain sufficient food for herself and her children.

Pearl: Karla paints houses with subsequent pain and discomfort in the UEs. Uninsured patients, particularly immigrants, frequently work in physically demanding jobs. As a result, they frequently experience joint, muscle, and back pain. If they are not educated or trained in other skills, they may not have a choice about where or how they work.

Mateo

Critical Thinking:

1) What are the major concerns in this case?

Tremors that are affecting Mateo's quality of life and ability to work. The patient cannot afford to see a neurologist.

Insomnia.

Left shoulder pain.

Hypertension—controlled.

Unknown maternal medical history.

Paternal medical history of colon cancer.

2) What is your plan for Mateo?

After obtaining standard labs and testing for autoimmune diseases (labs were normal except for lipids), the clinician brings Mateo back for a FU visit.

Due to the worsening of his tremors, the clinician decides to initiate a trial of Sinemet. She starts at a low dose of 10 mg/100 mg three times a day.

Refer Mateo for a colonoscopy; get a FIT in the meantime.

Start simvastatin 20 mg daily in the evening.

Suggest he try melatonin 3 mg for sleep.

3) What teaching is appropriate at this time?

Explain to Mateo that he displays some mild Parkinsonian symptoms that may be caused by an insufficient supply of a particular chemical in his body. The Sinemet will give him some of that chemical and should help if that is the reason for his tremors.

Instruct Mateo about a low-cholesterol, low-fat diet.

Mateo RTC for FU. He noticed a moderate decrease in tremors. The clinician increases the dose of Sinemet. On the subsequent visit, Mateo does not have any visible tremor and reports that he occasionally has a very slight tremor. He reports that his work has improved and he is able to remain employed.

> **Pearl:** In this case, it was possible to start the patient on a trial of medication that informed the clinician about the diagnosis based on the patient's response to the medication. This enabled the clinician to treat the patient without waiting for him to see a neurologist and an added expense. This was not a substitute for specialty care but was a temporary solution so Mateo could keep his job. Eventually, the clinician found a neurologist who was willing to see patients at a reduced cost and sent Mateo for a visit. There was no change in the diagnosis or treatment.

Natalia

Critical Thinking:

1) What are the major concerns in this case?
   Infection in finger.
   Needs preventive screening.
   Using condoms for birth control.
   Prediabetes.
   Depression and anxiety.
   Hyperlipidemia.
   Exposure of hands to water all day, daily.
2) What is your plan for Natalia?
   Treat infection.
   Give Natalia a note for work to not wash dishes for a few days so fingers can heal.
   Research, if possible, why Natalia had a mammogram at age 37. It may be appropriate to schedule a repeat mammogram.
   Schedule Pap smear.
3) What should be included in patient teaching for Natalia?
   Advise Natalia to wear long rubber gloves at work and to try to avoid getting water under gloves. Remove gloves regularly to dry hands and fingers. Apply lotion or petroleum jelly to hands at night and under gloves.
   Offer to discuss birth control options and explain that condoms are not as reliable as some other methods. Show Natalia pictures of birth control pill packs and IUDs and explain how they work.

> Pearl: Uninsured patients work in a variety of physically demanding occupations. Natalia washes dishes all day at a restaurant. Understanding that immigrants may have limited employment options, it is not helpful to recommend Natalia switch jobs. The clinician can serve her best by thinking creatively and recommending adjustments that might help the patient in her work.

Pedro

Critical Thinking:

1) What are the major concerns in this case?
   Pedro may lose his job because he is dropping things at work.

Chronic hand pain.

BL knee pain.

Nocturia ×4.

LE edema.

2) What is your plan for Pedro?

Blood work: UA, CBC, CMP, ANA with reflex, rheumatoid factor, CCP antibodies, ESR or CRP (it is too expensive to do both).

3) What teaching is appropriate at this time?

Use Voltaren gel to knee and hands prn pain. Only use ibuprofen or naproxen if gel or Tylenol does not relieve pain. Try heat to joints for relief. Elevate legs at the end of the day. Reduce soda intake; stop drinking liquids two hours before bedtime to reduce nocturia.

Pedro RTC two weeks later to review the laboratory results:

His blood work shows he is anemic. CMP is WNL.

ANA was negative. Rheumatoid factor, ESR, and CCP antibodies were abnormally elevated (CRP 5.57; ESR 86; RF 60.9). He reports that nocturia and other urinary symptoms have decreased.

Results of UA: blood +10; leukocytes 1+; nitrite positive; urobilinogen 2+; PH 6.0; specific gravity 1.020; protein +15; ketone negative; bilirubin 1+; glucose negative; color orange/clear.

On examination, he has left CVAT.

Pedro is asked to start Cipro 500 mg, 1 tablet, every 12 hours for 30 days and increase his water intake to 8 glasses per day. He is to start tamsulosin HCL 0.4 mg, 1 capsule, once a day. A renal ultrasound is ordered. A PSA is performed and is WNL. FIT is negative. A colonoscopy is ordered due to patient's age.

Critical Thinking:

1) How did the laboratory results refine the diagnosis?

Pedro has anemia of chronic disease.

He has rheumatoid arthritis.

He has prostatitis and BPH.

2) How will you choose affordable treatment for Pedro?

Unless a rheumatologist and urologist are available at reduced cost, the PCP must manage Pedro's care. The clinician consults a rheumatologist by phone to develop a plan. Pedro is asked to start methotrexate tablet, 2.5 mg, take six tablets once a week and folic acid tablet, 1 mg, once a day. He is asked to pick one day/week and take six tablets together on that day every week. The clinician explains that these medications are to resolve pain and prevent the rheumatoid arthritis from getting worse. They may take a few weeks to take effect. Pedro will need to have a CBC and CMP done every three months and RTC every three months for FU visits. He is to refrain from alcohol. He may take meloxicam 7.5 mg, one to two tablets per day, if has severe pain. The clinician can also order prednisone tablets to take if he has a flare. With a CRP of 5.57, Pedro is at high risk of a cardiac event, so he is started on ASA 81 mg/day.

Pedro obtains his lab work every three months and RTC every three months for a FU:

HPI: He states he feels much better and has no complaints. He reports morning stiffness of ½ hour to one hour and then "everything loosens up." He is taking methotrexate and folic acid as prescribed. He denies difficulty with medication tolerance. He denies urinary symptoms. Nocturia has decreased to once/night.

> Pearl: In this case, treatment made a big difference to Pedro's ability to work and keep his current employment. Pedro should be tested for *H. Pylori* and given omeprazole if he needs to continue taking an NSAID for pain.

Regina

Critical Thinking:

1) What are the major concerns in this case?
   Questionable adherence to medication regimen.
   Abnormal Pap smear three years ago.
   HTN.
   Obesity.
   Epigastric pain.
   Uterine prolapse and DUB.

Left foot pain.

Insomnia.

Hyperthyroidism.

2) What is your plan for Regina?

Pap smear.

TSH, T3, and T4 were abnormal.

BW: HgBA1C, CMP, CBC, lipid panel, UA, FIT (followed by colonoscopy when available).

Refer to podiatry.

Refer to gynecology.

Annual screening mammogram.

Monitor BP and treat as necessary.

3) What teaching is appropriate at this time?

Discuss sleep hygiene. Suggest Regina request regular shift hours and try to go to sleep at the same time every day. Explain that trazodone is not ideal for long-term treatment of insomnia. Unfortunately, cognitive behavioral therapy (CBT) is not available due to lack of insurance and the cost. Restricted sleep therapy is unlikely to work for her because her shifts change frequently.

Discuss the need to lose weight. Provide nutritional counseling. Discuss lowering intake of fat and carbohydrates and increasing fiber- and nutrient-rich foods, such as vegetables and fruit, fish, and nuts. She may need a multivitamin. Advise Regina to take calcium with vitamin D twice daily if she is not getting sufficient calcium through her diet. Alternatively, she can also take Tums with calcium plus a vitamin D3 tablet daily. This will give her sufficient calcium and help relieve acid reflux after it happens.

Review previous instructions with Regina regarding foods that can cause acid reflux. Remind her to take omeprazole daily.

Discuss footwear with Regina. She may not have access to podiatry, especially since she will have to pay for a visit to a gynecologist and for possible surgery. Give her exercises to do to stretch her feet and increase their strength. Encourage her to sit down if/when she gets a break at work.

Pearl: Regina works varying shifts for long hours, mostly standing. She works in food service so is exposed to fried and fatty food at work. It is difficult to treat insomnia in a patient with changing shifts who cannot take natural remedies such as melatonin or valerian root. Current best practices, such as sleep hygiene, CBT, and sleep restriction, may be unaffordable or unrealistic. The clinician who works with uninsured patients must frequently be prepared to counsel patients on topics for which they would typically refer patients to specialists. In this case, the clinician counsels Regina about sleep, foot wear, and nutrition. It is not uncommon to review several health concerns during one visit because it is difficult for many patients to RTC for FU as often as the clinician prefers. Patients may lose their jobs and frequently lose pay if they do not go to work. Most do not get vacation or sick time. The clinician must be sensitive to these concerns and be more flexible regarding televisits, prescription refills, and consults via phone without charge.

17

Trauma/Mental Health Issues

Alba

Critical Thinking:

1) What are the major concerns in this case?

Alba is alone in this country and has experienced several challenges: the death of her mother, an abusive boyfriend who is in jail, and financial difficulties.

Alopecia.

Forgetfulness.

Depression.

Obesity.

Prediabetes.

FMH of "kidney problems."

2) What is your plan for Alba?

BW results were all WNL, except for HgBA1C—6.2.

Start metformin HCL 500 mg, 1 tablet with a meal, once a day.

Refer to behavioral health.

Stress is probably contributing to alopecia and forgetfulness; however, Alba wears her hair drawn back tightly in a bun.

Provide nutritional counseling.

Refer her to county resources for financial assistance.

Research online or in-person groups that include people from Alba's country. These gatherings might provide support for her and help her to feel less isolated.

Caring for the Displaced and Uninsured: Clinical Case Studies in Nursing & Healthcare, First Edition. Leslie Neal-Boylan.
© 2023 John Wiley & Sons Ltd. Published 2023 by John Wiley & Sons Ltd.

Discuss birth control options when she is ready for a sexual relationship.

3) What patient teaching is appropriate at this time?

Tell Alba to take metformin with breakfast daily. Discuss starting a diabetic diet and provide written instructions. Discuss increasing exercise by walking daily. She should limit sugar and bread products, drink 8–12 glasses of water daily, and increase her intake of protein, fruits, and vegetables.

Alba refuses an antidepressant medication at this time.

Suggest Alba wear her hair less tightly and try taking biotin for her hair. Monitor HgBA1C because biotin can affect results.

> Pearl: Alba has experienced several challenges in her short life. She is alone in a new country without benefit of the language. She is already depressed. She will require social assistance and support beyond medical care.

Elena

Critical Thinking:

1) What are the major concerns in this case?

Obesity.

Needs preventive screening.

DMT2.

Hypertension.

Hyperlipidemia.

History of torture.

Loss of father and husband through homicide.

Unemployed.

Anxiety and depression.

2) What is your plan for Elena?

Elena is managing well with insulin and metformin. She denies signs or symptoms of hypoglycemia and is managing her diet. Her FBGs average 112 and her two-hour postprandial BGs average 135. She is due for BW: HgBA1C, CBC, CMP, albumin/creatinine ratio.

Elena's BP is well controlled with medication. Consider reducing the dose of losartan and rechecking BPs.

Screening mammogram.

Offer behavioral health counseling.

Spend time listening to Elena to try to understand her perception of her current situation.

3) What teaching is appropriate at this time?

Review diabetic diet, need for daily exercise, and weight loss. Explain what Elena's weight is using the BMI chart.

Explain that Elena's experiences might cause stress-related symptoms. Create an environment that helps her feel comfortable sharing her thoughts and concerns. Reassure her that the clinician and staff can help provide emotional support and direct her to resources that might help her.

Pearl: Not unlike many other immigrants, Elena has experienced torture and terrible loss. These experiences are worse than most Americans born in the United States can imagine or appreciate. It is important to listen and not try to normalize the patient's experiences or feelings. Platitudes are insulting and ineffective. Patients from other cultures may try to appear strong for caregivers, their children, and their employers, so others may not be aware of their continued emotional suffering and distress. It is necessary to provide a safe, unhurried environment for patients to talk if they want to and for the clinician to listen. Patients may not want, be able to afford, or have time for therapy. It is important to respect their reluctance to talk to others about their experiences.

Miguel

Critical Thinking:

1) What are the major concerns in this case?

Vision is changing.

Problems with his teeth.

LBP.

Physical job working as a painter and carpenter.

Three family members were murdered.

Worries about mother living in dangerous home country.

Hypertension.

Dry skin.

2) What is your plan for Miguel?

Lab work: CBC, CMP, HgBA1C, lipid panel, vitamin D, FIT and possible colonoscopy.

Give Miguel a flu shot and catch-up vaccines as needed and as affordable.

Refer Miguel for free vision and dental screening.

Manage his LBP with heat and NSAIDs, topical diclofenac gel.

Offer Miguel a note to rest from work for a few days.

Offer Miguel behavioral health if it can be obtained at low cost.

Offer Miguel information on the local food bank.

3) What teaching is appropriate at this time?

Ask Miguel to check his BP at a local pharmacy or grocery store two to three times per week and bring both the top and bottom numbers to the next visit. Teach him how to take his BP properly.

Advise him to use petroleum jelly to moisten skin. This is a cheap alternative to other creams and lotions.

Pearl: It is important to recognize that Miguel came to this country after tremendous hardship and loss. Be aware that he may consider health issues to be minor compared with what he has experienced and might not follow up or seek medical care when necessary. It is important to develop and maintain a relationship of trust so that he will feel comfortable returning to the clinic. Dental care beyond screening and cleaning can be very expensive and totally unaffordable for patients without insurance. Colonoscopy may also be unaffordable. Many patients, when asked to record their blood pressures, only record or remember the systolic number. It's important to educate them regarding how to monitor their blood pressure.

Darva

Critical Thinking:

1) What are the major concerns in this case?

Afraid to sleep.

Afraid she is going to die and that a witch is killing her.

Cannot work due to her fears and anxieties.

Alone in this country.

Darva is not eating much.

Needs vision, dental, and Pap smear screenings.

2) What is your plan for Darva?

Listening is most important during this and subsequent visits.

Complete physical exam today.

Standard blood work and urinalysis.

Evaluate whether Darva needs immediate inpatient care. If not, refer Darva to behavioral health as soon as possible.

Start Darva on sertraline 25 mg/day increasing to 50 mg/day after one week.

Start gabapentin 100 mg, 1–3 capsules at night to help her sleep until sertraline takes effect. Warn her of sleepiness during the day.

Discuss screenings at next visit.

3) What teaching is appropriate at this time?

Explain to Darva that a thorough PE and blood work will enable the clinician to find the cause of her symptoms.

Explain that a therapist can help Darva to talk through her worries and concerns.

Provide the crisis center hotline number so Darva can call someone anytime day or night if she is afraid.

Pearl: Patients from the United States or other countries may have superstitions that impact their perspectives on health. It is important to not disabuse patients of these beliefs until there is a strong rapport between the clinician and the patient. At such time, it may be helpful to have someone from behavioral health present or ask the person to have this conversation with the patient, especially if the therapist is from the same culture as the patient. Most importantly, the clinician must earn the patient's trust to treat. It may be possible to discuss the laboratory and examination results without discussing the superstitions if the patient accepts that the results may indicate why the patient is ill or having specific symptoms.

18

Specialty Access Issues

Carlos

Critical Thinking:

1) What are the major concerns in this case?
   Pt is visiting from his home country.
   It appears he was misdiagnosed in his home country.
   Carlos plans to stay in the United States.
   Carlos needs immediate, expensive care but has no insurance.
   He is not eligible for Medicaid.
   Carlos and his family are likely to have difficulty navigating the healthcare system.
2) What is your plan for Carlos?
   Support Carlos and his family.
   Find an oncologist willing to work with Carlos and his family and allow an installment payment plan. Some clinics have programs that can fund care for an eligible patient with urgent healthcare needs.
3) What patient teaching is appropriate at this time?
   Explain the diagnosis and what will likely happen next in the subsequent weeks and months. Remind the patient and family that the clinician is the PCP and will continue to be available for primary care concerns and questions.

Caring for the Displaced and Uninsured: Clinical Case Studies in Nursing & Healthcare, First Edition. Leslie Neal-Boylan.

Pearl: It is important to respect cultural and family practices. In this case, it was necessary to tell the son about the patient's diagnosis. The son then informed the patient. Then, both RTC to learn more about the diagnosis and next steps. In other cases, it may be necessary to speak to the patriarch of the family and have that person decide how best to inform the patient and family. In addition, Carlos has not had adequate access to healthcare until this point. As a result, his disease has advanced.

Sergio

Critical Thinking:

1) What are the major concerns in this case?
   Poor medication adherence.
   LE edema.
   Constipation.
   Dizziness.
   Poor water intake.
   HTN.
   DMT2.
2) What is your plan for Sergio?
   Increase fluid intake.
   BW: CBC, CMP, HgBA1C, lipids, UA, FIT (if unable to get lab results from NIH).
   Take one large spoonful of Metamucil with one large glass of water daily in the morning and increase overall fluid intake.
   Stop amlodipine.
   Add lisinopril 20 mg daily.
   Consider whether Sergio should continue taking aspirin daily.
3) What teaching is appropriate at this time?
   Review medications and the importance of taking them daily.
   Elevate legs when sitting.
   Avoid salt.

Sergio returns two months later:

HPI: Sergio presents for FU of dizziness, HTN, LE edema. He did not RTC for his two-week FU as requested. He states he feels well. He is only a little dizzy in the morning; this resolves as the day progresses. His son says that Sergio has been drinking more water. The LE edema resolved after stopping amlodipine. He has been taking his BP at home. The son says the systolic is 140, but he doesn't remember the diastolic reading. FBGs are running between 130 and 170 on glipizide 5 mg twice a day. Sergio denies chest pain, dyspnea, changes in mentation, or constipation.

Medications are refilled. Sergio is asked to check and record blood pressures two to three times each week: top and bottom numbers and heart rate. He is shown the correct way to measure blood pressure. He is started on atorvastatin 20 mg daily in the evening. He is asked to follow up in three months.

> Pearl: Participating in a clinical study is an option for uninsured patients to receive care and medications at no cost. However, this presents a few challenges for the clinician. The patient is being treated at two clinics; the patient may not be adherent to the study protocols unbeknownst to the researchers; it can be very difficult to find or reach a contact person directing the study or to obtain test results.

Sergio returns three months later:

HPI: Sergio RTC reporting lower abdominal pain and LE edema for two months. He resumed taking amlodipine daily. He also reports upper back pain for one month, constipation, BL knee pain, and occasional dyspnea.

Medications:

Metformin 1000 mg tablets, 1 tablet twice a day.
Amlodipine besylate 10 mg 1 tablet once a day.
Lisinopril 20 mg tablet, 1 tablet once a day.
Atorvastatin calcium 20 mg tablet, 1 tablet once a day.
Glipizide 10 mg 1 tablet in a.m. prebreakfast, 1 tablet in p.m. predinner.
Hydrochlorothiazide 25 mg, 1 tablet once a day.
Aspirin 81 mg, notes: 1 tablet qd.

ROS:

Endocrine: FBGs running 158–229 with average 178. Denies hypoglycemic symptoms. The patient reports he ran out of metformin.

Cardiovascular/respiratory: admits to shortness of breath at rest and with exertion. Admits to fluid accumulation in legs. Denies chest pain, dizziness, palpitations, cough, hemoptysis, pain with inspiration.

Gastrointestinal: admits to abdominal pain and swelling, constipation, heartburn. Denies blood in stool, diarrhea, nausea, vomiting.

Genitourinary: admits to frequent urination and nocturia ×2. Denies blood in urine or difficulty urinating.

Musculoskeletal: admits to BL knee pain and swelling, middle upper back pain. Denies recent falls.

Neurologic: denies tingling/numbness.

Vital Signs:

Ht 65 in, Wt 140 lbs, BP 140/76, HR 62/min, RR 16/min, Temp 98.5 F.

General Examination:

GENERAL APPEARANCE: alert, well hydrated, in no distress.

EYES: pupils equal, round, reactive to light and accommodation; a little difficulty with EOMs.

ORAL CAVITY: mucosa moist.

SKIN: warm and dry.

HEART: S1, S2 normal, regular rate and rhythm, no murmurs, rubs, gallops, no clicks.

LUNGS: clear to auscultation bilaterally.

ABDOMEN: R and L lower quadrant tenderness to palpation, no rebound, no masses palpable, no hepatosplenomegaly, no guarding or rigidity. No hernias.

BACK: TTP upper mid-back, normal exam of spine.

RECTAL: prostate is smooth but mildly enlarged, guaiac is negative.

EXTREMITIES: +4 pitting LE bilateral edema from knees to feet, good capillary refill in nail beds. No erythema, warmth, pallor, cold, pain, negative Homan's.

PERIPHERAL PULSES: 2+ dorsalis pedis, 2+ posterior tibial, 2+ radial.

NEUROLOGIC: nonfocal, alert and oriented.

Critical Thinking:

1) What are the major concerns in this case?
   Continued medication nonadherence.

Abdominal pain and distention.

BPH and urinary symptoms.

Dyspnea.

LE edema.

2) What is your plan for Sergio?

CXR.

Possible referral to cardiology.

Abdominal US.

Consider change of diuretic.

Stop amlodipine.

3) What teaching is appropriate at this time?

Call the clinic before you run out of medicine.

Review necessity for medication compliance.

Make FU appointment with NIH endocrinology—the patient may need assistance locating someone to contact.

Continue Metamucil fiber therapy daily.

Limit intake of liquids two to three hours before bedtime.

Use Tylenol for knee and back pain; may try OTC diclofenac gel for knee pain; also try heating pad.

Pearl: Patients may not always understand instructions, especially if English is not their first language. Patients are often eager to show they understand even if they do not. Interpreters may come from different countries and have regional accents or speak in an educated fashion to patients whom have not had any or minimal education. Patients may bring family members or friends to interpret for them, but these well-meaning people may not understand the instructions, especially if medical terminology is used. If possible, keep language simple and basic. Provide written materials in the patient's language.

Valeria

Critical Thinking:

1) What are the major concerns in this case?

Opioid use without a prescription.

Pelvic pain.

Left breast pain.

Fear of dying and leaving children alone.

Does not remember date of LMP.

2) What is your plan for Valeria?

The clinician will conduct a complete exam of the UEs.

Valeria likely has a leaking implant causing inflammation. She should continue applying warm compresses. The clinician will order pelvic and breast ultrasounds. While awaiting the results, the clinician will refer the patient to a breast surgeon because it can take months to get an appointment for an uninsured patient without breast cancer.

A urine pregnancy test will be obtained.

3) What patient teaching is appropriate at this time?

Instruct Valeria to avoid using prescriptions from other people and without a prescription. Encourage her to call the clinic for assistance and medication.

Valeria will be asked to record the dates of her periods and whether she has heavy or light bleeding and when. Following the pelvic ultrasound, the clinician will consider starting Valeria on OCPs to regulate her periods.

Valeria will be advised of the approximate cost of the breast surgeon visit so she can gather the necessary funds.

Pearl: Obtaining surgical consults and surgery is particularly challenging for uninsured patients. Surgery is expensive, and while surgeons might be willing to cut their price, costs remain for hospitalization, the room, anesthesia, medications, and care. After hospitalization or surgery, patients are often given discharge instructions to follow up with a specialist. The patient may not follow up due to the cost. If patients RTC with their PCP, the clinician may be able to arrange follow-up with a specialist at a reduced cost.

19

Delayed Screening

Aurora

Critical Thinking:

1) What are the major concerns in this case?
   Goiter.
   Last medical visit was five years ago.
   Due for Pap smear.
   Never had a mammogram.
   FMH of CVA.
   Peri-menopausal, not using birth control.
   High blood pressure.
2) What is your plan for Aurora?
   BW: CBC, CMP, HgBA1C, lipid panel, TSH, T4, and T3.
   Ultrasound of thyroid.
   Refer to endocrinology.
   RTC for Pap smear.
   Order mammogram.
   Refer for vision and dental screening.
3) What teaching is appropriate at this time?
   Explain to Aurora that it is important to keep up with regular/annual medical visits and preventive screening.
   Discuss contraceptive options.

Caring for the Displaced and Uninsured: Clinical Case Studies in Nursing & Healthcare, First Edition. Leslie Neal-Boylan.
© 2023 John Wiley & Sons Ltd. Published 2023 by John Wiley & Sons Ltd.

Ask Aurora to check her BP two to three times a week at a local pharmacy and to use the same pharmacy. Bring record to next visit.

Pearl: Uninsured patients may have missed preventive screening for a variety of reasons, such as lack of access to medical care in their home country, financial difficulties, lack of awareness of the necessity of preventive screening, fear (women may fear having pain during a mammogram or of what happens during a Pap smear), lack of understanding of how, where, or when to get screening and what screening is. The clinician can help by explaining the type of screening recommended and why. Mutual decision-making is key. Allowing patients a few visits to consider screening enables patients to feel they have choices and gives them multiple opportunities to ask questions and understand what is needed. They may talk to friends or family members between visits about their experiences with screening.

Mirikit

Critical Thinking:

1) What are the major concerns in this case?
   Mirikit has not had medical care for five years.
   She obtains her medicines from the Philippines, although she is not under the care of a provider.
   She takes vitamins although she has not been diagnosed with vitamin deficiencies.
   She had an abnormal Pap smear with no follow-up care.
   Her family medical history is unknown.
   She has a fibroid uterus.
   She works full time in a physical job.
2) What is your plan for Mirikit?
   Continue amlodipine.
   Increase valsartan to 80 mg.
   Order mammogram and pelvic ultrasound.

RTC for Pap smear.

BW: HgBA1C, CBC with differential/platelet, lipid panel, vitamin B12 and folate, vitamin D, 25-hydroxy, TSH, urinalysis.

Refer Mirikit for free vision and dental screening.

LDL is 160; HDL is 30.

Pap smear results: HGSIL, +HPV. A pelvic ultrasound reveals a large uterine fibroid.

3) What patient teaching is appropriate at this time?

Instruct Mirikit in the importance of regular and consistent medical care, monitoring of her blood pressure, and preventive screening. Explain that she should not be getting medications from the Philippines unless it has been prescribed. The clinician understands that she may not be able to afford medication in the United States. Explain that vitamins can be harmful if taken in large quantities when not needed. It is best to be tested for deficiencies before taking vitamins. Eating a healthful diet can preclude the need for vitamins in many instances. Mirikit should be assisted to understand the need for a repeat Pap smear and possibly a colposcopy, which will cost money. There may be a county program that can subsidize the procedure, if she qualifies. It is important to discuss the need for sufficient rest given Mirikit's physically taxing job. Mirikit is referred to a women's center for the uninsured for a colposcopy.

Mirikit presents for follow-up two weeks later:

HPI: She says she feels well. She has not heard about a GYN appointment yet. She had a vision screening and received a prescription for glasses. She has not yet had a dental screening. She occasionally checks her BP at home; systolic is in the 150s. She does not recall the diastolic.

Vital Signs:

BP 157/86 mmHg, HR 86/min, RR 16/min, Temp 98.6 F.

HCTZ 25 mg and simvastatin 20 mg are added to the regimen. She is encouraged to walk 30 minutes daily and eat a low-fat diet. She is given written information about a low-cholesterol, low-sodium diet. She is instructed in the importance of recording her BP three times/week and shown how to sit and rest prior to taking her BP. She is given a chart she can complete when she records her BP. She is to bring this to the next visit.

Mirikit RTC for FU in two weeks:

She had a colposcopy and was told she needs surgery, during which she will have the uterine fibroid removed. She states she prefers to wait until summer for the surgery because she is a housekeeper and babysits for work. In the summer, the parents of the children for whom she babysits can take vacation and watch the children while she has surgery and recuperates. Her BPs at home average 124/78.

The clinician explains that it is best for Mirikit to work out something with her employer so she can get the surgery soon because she has cervical cancer. The clinician offers to speak to the employer. Mirikit declines.

Pearl: Mirikit did not have a FU after an abnormal Pap smear. The repeat Pap was abnormal and likely worse than her previous abnormal Pap smear. The delay in screening was significant because Mirikit now needs surgery. An additional issue is the employer's reluctance to provide information necessary to show Mirikit's eligibility for a program that might help her get the necessary surgery. This might be viewed as exploitation of the patient by the employer, but the patient is reluctant to have the clinician advocate for her due to fear that she will lose her job.

20

Visitors

Franz

Critical Thinking:

1) What are the major concerns in this case?

   Franz is a visitor from Germany. He is highly educated and has insurance in his home country. He has kept current with his medical care.

   Needs medication refills; however, he did not bring any medical documentation to the visit.

   It is clear he has uncontrolled high blood pressure.

   Refuses blood work so it is difficult to ascertain his current state of health other than via patient report and physical examination.

   PMH of skin cancer.

   PMH of smoking.

   Drinks too much alcohol.

2) What is your plan for Franz?

   Refill lisinopril.

   The clinician is reluctant to refill sildenafil citrate without knowing Franz's cardiac history or laboratory results. Also, he is a smoker.

3) What patient teaching is appropriate at this time?

   Franz is encouraged to get lab tests, especially if he thinks he will remain in the United States for a prolonged period. Alternatively, he is asked to get copies of his medical visits and lab work from Germany.

Caring for the Displaced and Uninsured: Clinical Case Studies in Nursing & Healthcare, First Edition. Leslie Neal-Boylan.
© 2023 John Wiley & Sons Ltd. Published 2023 by John Wiley & Sons Ltd.

He is instructed to monitor his BP and regarding how to take his medications.

The clinician advises him to cut down on his alcohol intake.

The clinician reminds Franz to see his dermatologist annually.

Franz smoked for 20 years and quit 10 years ago so doesn't fit criteria for CT low-dose lung screening; however, he should confer with his primary care provider in Germany.

Pearl: Some patients may have insurance but be uninsured in the United States. Visitors who may be in the United States for prolonged periods may need medication refills or medical care. It is helpful if the visitors bring documentation of recent medical visits and test results when they seek a provider in the United States. However, if they do not, the clinician must start from scratch based on what the patient will allow and assume the patient is providing accurate information. Frequently, patients do not know the names of their medicines or their health conditions, as in the case of Marcos, below.

Marcos

Critical Thinking:

1) What are the major concerns in this case?

The patient needs medication refills but does not know names or dosages of his medications.

He is unable to get medical records from his home country.

FMH, including the type of cancer from which his mother died, is unknown.

HTN.

2) What is your plan for Marcos?

Marcos's son called back with the list of medications; however, if he was unable to obtain the names of the medications, Marcos would be advised to go to the ED to be evaluated and treated. He would have to pay for that visit. Following that visit, the clinic could use those medical records to treat the patient. The patient is told that it is unsafe to refill medications without knowing what they are.

3) What patient teaching is appropriate at this time?

Marcos should be instructed regarding the need to keep a record of his medications and dosages and a list of his medical conditions with him at all times.

He is advised of the need to RTC for a complete PE and laboratory analysis.

Pearl: It is not uncommon for patients to arrive at the clinic without the names or dosages of their medications. Frequently, the patient requires refills immediately. Consequently, the clinician has few choices but to ask the patient or family member to contact a family member in the home country to get the list of medications and diseases/conditions and convey that information to the patient over the phone, send the patient to the ED for immediate care, or start from scratch. Stat BW is expensive so the patient and clinician must wait until results return. Since Marcos had elevated BP in the clinic, the clinician could opt to start him on a low-dose antihypertensive available for free from the clinic samples. The patient can be asked to check his BP at a local grocery store pharmacy and RTC in one week with the record. This is not ideal but will give the clinician some idea of the patient's vital signs on a regular basis and the need for antihypertensive medications.

Trang

Critical Thinking:

1) What are the major concerns in this case?

Older adult visiting from Vietnam; wants to return to Vietnam.

Recent CVA.

Taking herbal medicines that may not be appropriate.

Hyperlipidemia.

HTN.

Family borrowing medicine and adjusting dosages.

Atherosclerosis, enlarged heart size.

Could benefit from additional home visits but cannot afford them.

2) What is your plan for Trang?
Review BW results from hospitalization.
Neurology consultation.
3) What teaching is appropriate at this time?
Explain to Trang and his son that Trang should not take any medications without discussing it with the clinician first. They should not adjust dosages without a discussion.
Explain that ginkgo biloba is a blood thinner, so it is best to discontinue it.
Trang is a self-pay patient. The clinician explains to his son that he needs to contact a neurologist and pay for the visit. The clinician gives him a list of local neurologists and their prices for an initial consult.
Explain that ginseng can raise or lower BP.
Explain that most function following a CVA is regained in the first six months. Trang is not ready to take a long trip to his home country.

Trang and his son RTC one week later for a follow-up visit:

HPI: Trang is wearing pajamas under his raincoat. He states he feels better, although he felt very tired yesterday and rested all day. He received a home visit from the ST that helped with drinking and swallowing. He has had one visit from OT. PT came to the home but was unable to work with the patient because Trang's BP was high. Trang reports he is sleeping well but has nocturia three to four times nightly. The commode is next to the bed. He is using the walker at home but is not walking much. He mostly sits on the couch in the living room. BPs at home range in the evening from 132/82, pulse 68, to 170/92, pulse 66. He is taking lisinopril 20 mg daily in the morning. The son has not yet made an appointment with a neurologist.

General Examination:

GENERAL APPEARANCE: unremarkable.NEUROLOGIC: better this visit. Trang is able to identify the day of the week, the month, and the year. He is able to describe why he is in clinic today.
The clinician decides to add amlodipine 5 mg to be taken at night. Trang is to continue taking lisinopril in the evening, aspirin in morning, and rosuvastatin at night. Trang is asked to stop using ginseng

until the next visit. The son is asked to continue recording the BP, one to two hours after the evening medicine. Trang should avoid using salt in his food. The clinician explains to Trang's son that Trang should be walking with the walker frequently throughout the day. He should dress daily and participate in normal activities—with supervision. He should not be in bed or lie down all day. Trang needs to regain his strength; activity is also better for his mental health. Trang should not be cooking and he is not to be left alone or unsupervised. Trang is advised to stop drinking fluids two hours before bedtime to reduce nocturia.

Trang and his son follow up in two weeks:

Trang is doing well. His BPs have normalized. He is taking his medications as prescribed. Nocturia has decreased to twice per night. He is encouraged to increase activity, as tolerated, and continue when he is outside to use the walker to prevent falls. He has an appointment with PT next week at home. The son has not yet contacted neurology for an appointment.

Trang and his son have several telehealth visits before they RTC in person six months later:

Trang is walking steadily independently but still uses the walker when he goes to a store with his son. He is dressed appropriately in a suit that has been pressed. He makes eye contact and is alert and oriented ×4. He says he feels "great." He wants to go home to Vietnam. Trang's son says they have made arrangements for another son to travel with Trang. Flights have been split up over two days; each flight is approximately eight hours. Trang will sleep in a hotel overnight between flights. Trang and his son verbalize understanding that Trang will be sure to take all his medications including aspirin and to keep in mind the time change when taking his medications The clinician explains that Trang should wear compression hose, walk in the airplane aisles at least once every hour, and pump his feet and ankles frequently while sitting. The son has already scheduled Trang for an appointment within the week of his arrival home with his medical provider in Vietnam. He is given copies of the hospital notes, progress notes, and lab and radiology results to take with him to show his provider.

Pearl: Patients who are visiting the United States frequently intend to go home; however, others may choose to stay. Patients with serious health conditions require some preparation before making a long trip back to their home country. Clinicians are responsible for understanding where patients plan to go, how, and with whom so they can help the patient develop the necessary strength and endurance to travel. This also applies to patients who are going home for a visit. They may not be able to get to a medical provider right away once they reach their destination so may need medications for three months. It is also important to help patients and families understand how challenging and tiring travel is for a person who is not well and/ or elderly and that a medical appointment should be arranged ahead of time to occur shortly after arrival. Patients may think they can ask the provider in the United States to continue to supply them with medications while they are out of the country. It is helpful to the provider at the destination if the clinician in the United States sends the patient with copies of recent progress notes and test results.

21

Immigration Issues

Gabriela

Critical Thinking:

1) What are the major concerns in this case?
Patient spent one year in an immigration detention center.
Possible hypothyroidism; unsure of medication dose.
Not taking any medication.
Cannot afford food.
Far away from her children.
Depression, anxiety, insomnia.
Hair loss.
Weight loss.
Needs eye exam and to see a dentist.
Not using birth control (husband is in home country, but she says she is sexually active).
Needs Pap smear.
Epigastric pain with unintentional weight loss.
2) What is your plan for Gabriela?
Gabriela needs a complete PE and BW: CBC, CMP, HgBA1C, lipid panel, TSH, UA.
She may need catch-up immunizations.
It is not known if Gabriela will RTC for FU so the clinician decides to start her on low-dose levothyroxine.
Refer her to local food banks and to county emergency assistance.

Caring for the Displaced and Uninsured: Clinical Case Studies in Nursing & Healthcare, First Edition. Leslie Neal-Boylan.

Refer to behavioral health.

Refer for free vision screening and give her names of dentists who speak Spanish.

Consider starting Gabriela on a PPI, such as omeprazole, daily.

3) What teaching is appropriate at this time?

Provide diet information and nutritional counseling with the understanding that Gabriela is currently eating what she can access and afford. That food is likely fast and/or fried food. This is probably contributing to her epigastric pain. However, anxiety may also be a contributor.

Suggest Gabriela use condoms whenever involved in sexual activity with men; however, it is important to clarify if she is only sexually active with her husband, either when she is in her home country or when he is visiting her in the United States, and whether she wants to get pregnant. If not, she will need a more reliable form of birth control.

Pearl: Unless the patient brings papers from the immigration detention center (not typical), the clinician will not have any information about what happened there from a medical perspective. Many patients from other countries have not had childhood or adult immunizations and some may have been given COVID-19 vaccines that are not approved in the United States. It is likely the latter would have been corrected at the detention center; however, the patient may not have had other vaccines.

Isabella

Critical Thinking:

1) What are the major concerns in this case?

Isabella probably has PTSD from violence experienced in her home country.

Insomnia r/t anxiety and getting up with an infant.

Isabella is lactating but is taking an unknown medication that may be harmful to her infant.

Missed period and BL pelvic pain.

No birth control (but currently has no partner).

Needs vision and dental screening.

Unemployed without partner to help with finances or children.

2) What is your plan for Isabella?

Lab work: CBC, CMP, HgBA1C, lipid panel, TSH, UA.

Urine pregnancy test; result is negative. Isabella is started on Nora-BE 0.35 mg, 1 tablet, once a day.

Refer for free vision and dental screening.

Start sertraline, which is considered safe during lactation. Start with 25 mg every day for one week, then increase it to 50 mg daily.

Refer Isabella to behavioral health.

3) What teaching is appropriate at this time?

Explain that Isabella should not take medications without consulting the clinician, especially since she is breastfeeding. She should stop current antianxiety medication and start sertraline.

Offer information regarding housing, financial assistance, and food banks.

Pearl: Isabella has experienced violence in her country, and despite being in the United States and feeling safe in her home, she still feels very anxious about her safety and that of her children. She is living with her parents, but it is up to her to assist them as they navigate the intricacies of being in the United States and not speaking the language. She has responsibilities to her parents and her children without any support. It is important to provide her with resources and help her overcome language barriers to get what she needs.

Ivanna

Critical Thinking:

1) What are the major concerns in this case?

Ivanna is a young woman who walked alone through several countries to reach the United States.

She is living alone in a shelter.

She is working part time in a physical job: house cleaning.

She has pain in BL wrists and bases of thumbs.

She is a smoker.

She needs glasses because hers broke.

Low back pain; obesity.

Excessive alcohol use.

Amenorrhea for four months.

Alopecia.

Parents' medical history is unknown.

2) What is your plan for Ivanna?

Pregnancy test.

BW: CBC, CMP, HgBA1C, lipid panel, TSH, ANA with reflex, rheumatoid arthritis factor, sedimentation rate, CCP antibodies IgG/IgA, UA.

All adult patients should be tested for HIV and hepatitis B and C. This can be done at a later visit.

Flu shot; consider catch-up immunizations. Offer information regarding COVID-19 vaccinations.

Refer for free vision and dental screening.

Continue naproxen, 250 mg, 1 tablet with food or milk, twice a day.

X-ray of bilateral wrists.

Consider EMG and nerve conduction studies at a later visit; however, these are very expensive without insurance.

Offer a note for work to refrain from using her hands for a couple of days.

3) What patient teaching is appropriate at this time?

It is necessary to prioritize Ivanna's treatment plan and hope she will RTC for continued patient education.

The clinician explains that a combination of stress and having been on Depo-Provera likely caused amenorrhea. She advises Ivanna that OCPs might be her best option to regulate her periods, or she can go to Planned Parenthood for an IUD. This discussion is best left to the next visit. For now, the clinician recommends using condoms to prevent pregnancy and STIs.

The clinician explains that strenuous activity, such as her migration and working as a house cleaner, can contribute to back and joint pain. The lab work will determine whether she has an autoimmune condition that might be causing her symptoms.

Suggest that, for now, Ivanna continue to wear the wrists splints at night. Drink 8–12 glasses of water/day to prevent constipation from naproxen.

Advise Ivanna that she can get reading glasses at any local pharmacy and that the optometrist at the vision screening will give her a prescription for other glasses, if she needs them.

Suggest that Ivanna reduce alcohol and tobacco use but save an in-depth discussion for the next visit.

Pearl: Many patients emigrate to the United States via hardship and physically taxing efforts. Ivanna has experienced a lot of stressful events that may be the causes of her health concerns. She requires reassurance and support. The clinician must spend time listening and empathizing. Sometimes, patients need incentives to RTC for continued care. Patients benefit from a trusting relationship with the clinician and the perception that someone truly cares for their welfare and success in their new country.

Junior

Critical Thinking:

1) What are the major concerns in this case?
   Right knee pain and swelling.
   Had to flee home country.
   HTN.
   LE edema.
   Needs dental screening.
   ED.
   Acid reflux.
2) What is your plan for Junior?
   Consider imaging for knee if NSAIDs are ineffective.
   BP management.
   Refer for free dental screening.
   Prescribe Viagra 25 mg prn ED.
3) What teaching is appropriate at this time?
   Take BP medications properly and daily.
   Exercise 30 minutes daily.
   Avoid spicy and fried food; avoid heavy meals, reduce coffee intake.
   Sit up for 30 minutes after eating.

This patient required several visits to adjust his medication to protect his kidney function and improve his BP. He was able to see a nephrologist working at another clinic for the uninsured. The clinician discontinued amlodipine and his LE swelling resolved. Carvedilol was also discontinued. He was started on Accupril. He continued to have OA in his knees. He used honey topically with relief.

Pearl: It is not unusual to have patients who have fled their home countries due to political turmoil, murders of friends or family members, torture, violence, or threats to their safety. Some patients lose their livelihood. It can be painful for patients to be in the United States and have family "back home." Sometimes they feel they have abandoned their families and friends, especially if parents arrive first and bring their children once they are settled. It is difficult for many adults to get employment in the United States, especially if they are older. Educated, professional people who have fled to the United States must frequently take menial jobs to feed themselves and their families.

22

Other

Julio

Critical Thinking:

4) What are the major concerns in this case?
   BPH.
   History of kidney stones.
   Dysuria.
   Hemorrhoid and condyloma acuminata.
   Anxiety.
   Alcohol use disorder.
   Uses marijuana.
   Flatulence and abdominal pain.
   Obtaining prescriptions and medical care long distance.
5) What is your plan for Julio?
   BW; Julio refuses because he says his provider in his country "already did that and everything was fine."
   UA.
   Offer renal ultrasound; Julio refuses.
   Order Anusol cream for external hemorrhoid.
   Order a FIT.
   Explore whether Julio has chronic or acute anxiety with possible referral to behavioral health.
   Explore Julio's diet; consider a trial of simethicone tablets for flatulence.

Caring for the Displaced and Uninsured: Clinical Case Studies in Nursing & Healthcare, First Edition. Leslie Neal-Boylan.
© 2023 John Wiley & Sons Ltd. Published 2023 by John Wiley & Sons Ltd.

6) What teaching is appropriate at this time?

Help Julio understand that his intake of alcohol is excessive and can damage the liver and cause chronic disease. Offer support group resources, if available at low cost. Explain that marijuana can affect the lungs and be detrimental to his health.

Explain the causes of hemorrhoids and recommend that Julio take a fiber supplement daily with a large glass of water to prevent hard stools.

Instruct Julio regarding condyloma acuminata: causes and prevention. The clinician explains that there is treatment, but they can also be left alone if they are not bothering Julio. However, condyloma acuminata are sexually transmitted and may take years to go away without treatment.

Explain to Julio that the clinician cannot prescribe for another provider from another country. Julio did not bring any documentation of visits or lab results. He explains that it is necessary to conduct his own exam and obtain lab results to understand Julio's current state of health. The clinician also explains that the 24-hour urine test is expensive. However, the clinician agrees to order the 24-hour urine. The clinician declines to order another medication for Julio's BPH or urinary symptoms (the UA was negative).

Pearl: It is not uncommon for patients to continue to work with someone from their own country and with whom they feel most comfortable. These telehealth visits are frequently free. This presents a challenge for the clinician both from a medical perspective and to incentivize the patient to RTC. Flexibility is often required. In this case, Julio is willing to pay for the 24-hour urine test and there is no harm in ordering it. His history and symptoms justify the order. This flexibility would probably not be possible in a private practice.

Mario

Critical Thinking:

1) What are the major concerns in this case?

Chest pain with history of acid reflux.

Never had medical exam, vision or dental screening.

Left LE pain.

BL foot pain.

Stands all day at work.

Smoker ×28 years.

Lives in a basement.

Medical history of parents is unknown.

Mario does not read or write in any language.

2) What is your plan for Mario?

Order a CT of the chest (28-year history of smoking).

Order an EKG now.

Refer for free vision and dental screening.

Order a PPI to be taken ½ hour before breakfast. Mario should stop taking his current OTC med for acid reflux of unknown name.

Refer Mario to a podiatrist if available and for reduced cost. Suggest Mario consider buying new shoes. His may be worn out.

Suggest NSAIDs for LE and foot pain.

Consider a trial of gabapentin for "shooting" pain.

Ensure Mario has access to sufficient and nutritious food and feels safe in his environment.

3) What patient teaching is appropriate at this time?

Praise Mario for maintaining smoking cessation and explain why he needs a CT. This may have to be postponed until Mario can afford to get the CT. The clinician might order a chest x-ray in the meantime.

Ask Mario to stop taking the medicine he is taking at home or to have a family member or friend call the clinic to tell the clinician the name of the medication. Discuss dietary changes that might reduce acid reflux. Instruct Mario to go to the ED if chest pain persists/worsens despite taking the PPI. Encourage Mario to use a block of wood to raise the head of the bed 6–12 inches. Encourage him to sit up for at least 30 minutes after eating, to eat and chew slowly, and to avoid laughing or talking while eating.

Teach Mario correct techniques for bending and lifting.

Instruct Mario on exercises he can perform for plantar fasciitis; suggest he freeze a bottle of water and roll his foot over it when he has pain. Provide stretching instructions with pictures for plantar fasciitis.

Pearl: It is not unusual for immigrant patients to be unable to read or write in their own language. Showing patients pictures on the computer screen can help them understand their condition and their treatment. Many patients have cell phones and can take photos of the pictures on the computer screen. The clinic should also have written instructions in English and other languages. It is also common for BPs to be elevated in the clinic but not at home. While this is also true for insured patients, uninsured patients may be particularly anxious because they have never had a medical visit, it has been a very long time since a medical visit, or this is the first medical visit in the United States.

Ramon

Critical Thinking:

1) What are the major concerns in this case?
    S/P hospitalization.
    Alcohol and cocaine intoxication; substance use disorder.
    Acute hepatitis.
    Use of medications without a prescription.
    Hypertension.
    Rhabdomyolysis.
    Toothache, poor dentition.
    Abdominal pain, nausea, chills.
    Unemployed.
    Smoker.
    Obesity.
2) What is your plan for Ramon?
    BW: CBC, CMP, lipid panel, HgBA1C, UA, CK.
    Assist Ramon to find affordable resources for support for substance use disorder. Support Ramon in his effort to maintain abstinence.
    Consult a gastroenterologist regarding next steps.
    Refer Ramon to behavioral health, if available.
    Encourage Ramon to get tested for HIV and STIs.
    Ramon needs close follow-up.

Refer Ramon to a dentist if available and affordable; treat his dental pain with analgesics and comfort measures.

3) What teaching is appropriate at this time?

Educate Ramon about the harm caused by excessive Tylenol, the use of medications without prescriptions, and opioid use. Discuss the potential for harmful interactions of medications, especially when also adding alcohol. Explain that Ramon should avoid getting medications from the Latin store. Rather, he should come to or call the clinic about medication prescriptions and use.

Educate Ramon about what "fatty liver" means and how weight loss can reduce fatty liver. Explain how medications and alcohol can also damage the liver and why that is bad.

Instruct Ramon in the importance of taking his medications as prescribed. Explain that the nausea is likely to subside as his body continues to recover.

Explain that the effects of PCP in the body are very similar to the effects from cocaine.

Educate Ramon about the effects of tobacco; suggest over the course of several visits that he cut down. This may need to wait until he recovers from his recent hospitalization and is able to cut down on drug and alcohol use.

Pearl: Ramon's case is an example of a patient who may appear as a new patient posthospitalization and may never have had medical care or has not had medical care for many years. Ramon was treated but did not RTC for FU. Some patients, such as Ramon, RTC every year or so for medication if they feel they need it or it has helped them. Working with them often requires starting all over again to assess their current health status and determine their needs. Typically, BW requires repeating and a complete PE is necessary. It is not uncommon for patients like Ramon to go back to the hospital or a rehabilitation facility on multiple occasions and be told to FU with primary care. This establishes a cycle of starting "fresh" each visit and an inability to make progress in the patient's treatment. Online resources that list data and documentation and from hospitalizations and urgent care visits are invaluable in these cases.

Conclusion

The cases within this book illustrate the continued disparities in health care based on race, ethnicity, citizenship, and financial status. People without insurance are frequently bereft of adequate resources to meet their health care needs. Patients who pay out of pocket can rarely afford to see specialists, have surgery, or pay for specialized testing. People with Medicare or Medicaid have greater access in some respects, but not all clinics take these patients. In a clinic focused on the uninsured, patients with Medicare or Medicaid cannot access the resources reserved for people without any insurance. They must find their own specialists and hope they take Medicare or Medicaid.

It is ironic that uninsured patients in a community clinic should frequently receive more time and attention than patients in private clinics. Managed care and the regulations that have evolved over the last three or four decades have necessitated very short primary care visits, limits on tests that can be ordered, and specialty referrals. Clinics for the uninsured (they vary, so this might not hold true for all of them) have the luxury of ignoring these requirements because their patients do not have insurance. While there is motivation to see as many patients as possible in a day because patients often pay a fee, albeit a low fee, providers are not restricted to the same degree regarding how much time they spend with patients, how many health concerns they address, or whether they order tests or medications they deem necessary but are not approved by insurance companies. While it is vital that all clinicians adhere to standards of care and clinical guidelines, these are interpreted based on

Caring for the Displaced and Uninsured: Clinical Case Studies in Nursing & Healthcare, First Edition. Leslie Neal-Boylan.
© 2023 John Wiley & Sons Ltd. Published 2023 by John Wiley & Sons Ltd.

the individual patient and the patient's past medical history and financial wherewithal.

These community clinics are at a disadvantage because of financial constraints; however, clinicians have the opportunity, in many cases, to practice medicine as it was meant to be practiced by treating patients' holistic needs, having time to talk with patients, and getting to know patients and their significant others. The primary care clinician in this setting is able to combine traditional, allopathic medicine with safe treatments valued by other cultures. Frequently, treatment must resort to the basics because anything beyond that is unaffordable. However sometimes the basics are all that anyone needs: rest, fluids, a mild analgesic, and the comfort of home and loved ones. Pharmaceutical companies have drawn providers away from the basics, encouraging us to prescribe tests and treatments that may be unnecessary. Without the temptation to order a lot of tests or prescribe expensive medications, clinicians must seek other ways of diagnosing and treating patients with the same high standard of care.

It has long been apparent that policy changes are required to manage the costs of medications, insurance, and health care. Dental insurance, even when available, provides scant coverage beyond dental cleaning. The health of the teeth is vital to overall health and wellness. I am not a politician or a policy maker so am not in a position to propose specifics of policy changes; however, it is clear the United States needs AFFORDABLE, HIGH-QUALITY, EQUITABLE health care for all. It is a right, not a privilege.

Index